cardiac
rehabilitation

cardiac rehabilitation:
a comprehensive nursing approach

Patricia McCall Comoss, R.N., CCRN
Senior Nursing Consultant
Nursing Enrichment Consultants, Inc.
Harrisburg, Pa.

E. Ann Smith Burke, R.N., CCRN
Formerly Instructor Rehab Hospital Educational Department
Harrisburg, Pa.

Susan Herr Swails, R.N.
Cardiac Rehabilitation Nurse Specialist
Cardiac Treatment Center, Holy Spirit Hospital
Camp Hill, Pa.

J. B. Lippincott Company
Philadelphia   New York   Toronto

ISBN 0-397-54322-0

Library of Congress Catalog Card Number 79-13050

Printed in the United States of America

2   4   6   8   9   7   5   3   1

Library of Congress Cataloging in Publication Data

Comoss, Patricia McCall.
  Cardiac rehabilitation.

  Includes bibliographical references and index.
  1. Cardiovascular disease nursing. 2. Cardiovascular patient—Rehabilitation. I. Burke, E. Ann Smith, joint author. II. Swails, Susan Herr, joint author.
  III. Title. [DNLM: 1. Heart diseases—Rehabilitation —Nursing texts. WY152.5 C735c]
RC674.C64   610.73′6   79-13050
ISBN 0-397-54322-0

dedication

This book is dedicated to
R. A. Ortenzio
who brought us together
and gave us a chance

and to
the nearly 300 cardiac rehab
nurse pioneers with whom
we learned and grew

preface

That the practice of nursing is undergoing change is not news. That cardiac care has evolved from an acute specialty to include preventive and rehabilitative emphasis is not news. That the 1970s have witnessed the entwining of these two events *is* news to cardiac patients and health care professionals alike. The result of this modern merger is that more and more nurses are practicing expanded professional roles in cardiac rehabilitation settings.

Textbooks abound on expanded roles in nursing. But in over eight years of practice and teaching in the developing field of cardiac rehabilitation, the authors have repeatedly recognized the lack of related nursing texts. This book is our endeavor to fill the void on nurses' bookshelves with a comprehensive volume on the professional nurse's role in cardiac rehabilitation.

The framework for the book is provided by the practice model presented in the Introduction. Each unit of the text corresponds to a phase of cardiac rehabilitation. Chapters within each unit define the nurse's role according to components of the nursing process.

Every chapter begins with a list of behavioral objectives. Intended as learning guides, the objectives indicate what the reader should be able to do following completion of the chapter to reflect that learning has been accomplished.

Text content describes prevailing theories and provides practical considerations. A sample case is used throughout to illustrate the nursing functions discussed in the preceding pages.

The authors feel that this structure offers several advantages to the intended readership. First, the nurse generalist and the primary care nurse interested in the theories and principles of cardiac rehabilitation nursing should find the sequential presentation logical and easy to read. Second, the nurse specialist practicing in a specific rehabilitation setting will be able to isolate and intensify the rehab segment of interest to her. Third, the nurse educator can select independent parts of the text appropriate for teaching needs. Fourth, nurses, nursing students, and other health care professionals interested in cardiac rehabilitation will find the format useful for quick and easy reference.

Although comprehensive in its nursing practice descriptions, this book is not a primer on basic cardiac care. In fact, Unit I begins where most cardiac care books end—with the acute coronary patient stabilized in CCU, a coronary care unit. Chapter 20 fades with the same coronary patient one year later, doing more and enjoying more than ever before. The how's and why's of this modern transformation span all the chapters in between.

The authors would like to express their awareness that both women and men practice nursing and that both women and men have cardiac disease. However, constant repetition of the descriptive nouns "nurse" and "patient," as well as use of the double pronoun he/she presented writing and reading impediments. Therefore, based on population majority in our nursing experience, we have elected to use the pronoun "she" when speaking of the nurse and the pronoun "he" when discussing the patient.

acknowledgments

No author, or group of authors, can be all things to a work in progress. We are no exception. Without the assistance of the following people, the finished product would not have become a reality. We are grateful to:

Our Nurse Editors:

Expert critical care and cardiac rehab specialists who helped us to see and hear what we were writing and to maintain our perspective.

Frances E. Burkholder, R.N., M.S.
Jerlynn B. Gruber, R.N., CCRN, B.S.
Donna M. Havens, R.N., B.S.
Angela D. Lehman, R.N.
Ruth A. Matthews, R.N.
Margaret McCall, R.N.
A. Ellen Sartori, R.N.

Our Teacher Editors:

Experts on the written word without whose translation we would not have been able to say what we meant.

Alicia M. McCall, B.S.
Daniel R. Shaffer, B.S.
Kathryn A. Walsh, B.S., M.Ed.

Our Special Interest Editors:

Experts not only in their respective fields but also in their ability to relate to broader health interests.

Richard L. Coulson, M.Sc., Ph.D.
Robert L. Jones, M.S., D.Ed.
James D. McCall, R.Ph.

The Nursing Staff of the Cardiac Rehabilitation Center, Rehab Hospital, Mechanicsburg, Pennsylvania:

Cardiac rehab specialists who shared their nursing experiences and patient data so we all could learn.

Jacquelyn F. Kreitzer, R.N.
Roxanne L. Stoner, R.N.
Vivian Wisniewski, R.N.

R. Lynn McGuire

For sharing a part of himself.

Lynne R. Rickenbach

For dedication and deligence far beyond the call of duty.

Nanette K. Wenger, M.D.

For all she has taught us, for her comments on this project, and especially for her continuing inspiration.

and to

David T. Miller and the J. B. Lippincott Company

For this experience!

foreword

One of the most exciting features of the rehabilitative approach to the patient with symptomatic coronary disease has been its progressive incorporation into the mainstream of traditional medical care. Additionally, the multidisciplinary approach to rehabilitation enables more effective and complete restoration of the patient to an optimal functional level in a variety of spheres: physiological, psychological, social, educational, vocational.

Nursing roles within the health care team may vary considerably, depending on the size of the patient population served, the scope and mode of organization of rehabilitation services, the extent of participation of the other health care disciplines in the rehabilitation team, the community medical practice customs, and so on. This text admirably serves the educational needs of the rehabilitation nurse in reviewing a variety of rehabilitation-related activities and programs both during the acute care (in-hospital) and the convalescent-recovery (posthospital) phases of myocardial infarction. It reflects both the scientific and the practice-related expertise of the authors.

The background information offers a comprehensive review, with appropriate references selected for the reader who wishes to explore an area in greater depth. Definition of the behavioral objectives for each chapter not only summarizes the cognitive and performance skills necessary for a rehabilitation nurse, but enables self-assessment of the adequacy of factual and programmatic material derived from the chapter. Serial application of the nursing process: assessment, planning, implementation and evaluation—can be equally well utilized by other members of the rehabilitation team, for whom this text is also recommended, because of the overlapping and varying professional roles in many hospital and community rehabilitation programs.

Review of this text will also enable the coronary care nurse or "generalist" nurse caring for coronary patients to gain insight into the rehabilitative approach and thus be better able to re-enforce its goals and its implementation.

The authors have made an important contribution to the care of patients with symptomatic coronary atherosclerotic heart disease, this nation's most prevalent health problem.

Nanette Kass Wenger, M.D.
Professor of Medicine (Cardiology)
Emory University School of Medicine
Director—Cardiac Clinics
Grady Memorial Hospital
Atlanta, Georgia

contents

introduction:
a philosophy and
a model for nursing
practice in cardiac
rehabilitation

Cardiac rehabilitation may be defined as the process of actively assisting the known cardiac patient to achieve and maintain his optimal state of health. Words used in this definition were chosen specifically to connote certain beliefs that the authors feel are essential to meaningful nursing care in a cardiac rehabilitation setting.

". . . the process of actively assisting . . ."

Rehabilitation is accomplished by the patient, not administered by the nurse. The desire to accomplish rehabilitation goals must be intrinsic. The nurse cannot give the patient motivation in a capsule. However, if patient and nurse work together, identifying problems and planning solutions, the partnership can provide the assistance and support necessary to reach mutual goals.

". . . the known cardiac patient . . ."

Ideally, cardiac rehabilitation begins at the time a diagnosis of coronary artery disease is made. Such diagnosis is usually the result of an acute event, often a myocardial infarction, which is like a neon sign flashing attention to the underlying catastrophe of coronary artery disease.

Although the authors realize that other types of cardiac disease require rehabilitative care, this text will focus on patients with coronary artery disease. The postmyocardial infarction patient will be used to typify the needs and processes of cardiac rehabilitation.

". . . to achieve and maintain . . ."

Two active verbs are included in the goal statement to designate both short- and long-term purposes of cardiac rehabilitation. To simply reach a predefined goal does not complete the rehabilitation process. Continuing healthful habits as an important part of everyday life is the long-term objective. Since cardiac rehabilitation belongs to the patient, it should not end when he departs the protective custody of his nurse.

Although a frequent word in definitions of rehabilitation, the authors have chosen not to use the noun "restoration" or its verb form "to restore." Phraseology related to restoration is frequently misinterpreted to mean the return of the patient to his preacute health state. Due to the insidious nature of coronary artery disease, a preacute state may be functional, but is obviously not healthful.

". . . optimal state of health . . ."

The optimal state for a given patient is one which is most effective for and most meaningful to him. It does not necessarily represent the pinnacle of his capabilities, and, therefore, the term "maximal" would be inappropriate. Identifying this optimal position is part of the goal-setting that will be done by the patient with support and assistance from his rehab nurse.

As defined by the World Health Organization, health is ". . . the state of complete physical, mental, and social well-being, and not merely the absence of disease or infirmity."[1] In cardiac rehabilitation, the existence of coronary artery disease is acknowledged and accepted. It is known from the start that the rehabilitation process will not "cure" the pathology. Awareness that a high level of well-being can be attained in spite of the disease may be the primary motivation for both patient and nurse.

Cardiac rehabilitation, as seen in the preceding definition, is a complex undertaking. It has been described as a subdiscipline of cardiology, which has introduced many innovative approaches for care of the cardiac patient.[2]

Cardiac rehabilitation is not the sole responsibility of a single health profession. In its simplest form it requires cooperation and collaboration between physician and nurse. Large formal rehabilitation programs may include any number of health professionals, such as dietitians, pharmacists, physical therapists, occupational therapists, exercise physiologists, vocational rehabilitation counselors, psychologists, social workers, and more. Regardless of the number of people involved, the patient remains the most important member of the rehab "team."

It is the authors' opinion that the nurse's role in any cardiac rehabilitation setting is of major importance. As the health professional spending most of her time in direct patient contact, the nurse should assume responsibility for much of the rehab process.

Depending upon the nursing philosophy of an institution and upon specific nursing positions, the job description of a cardiac rehab nurse will vary somewhat. In some hospitals, the patient's primary care nurse will assist with cardiac rehabilitation. In others, a nurse specialist is assigned to rehab functions. And in still others, rehabilitation is the responsibility of the general nursing staff. Whatever the actual job description, the nurse in a cardiac rehabilitation setting becomes a "coordinator" of rehab care, assessing the patient's health needs, planning and implementing appropriate interventions, and evaluating rehab effectiveness. This emerging professional role is in keeping with the Standards of Cardiovascular Nursing Practice as adopted by the American Nurses' Association and American Heart Association.[3]

Cardiac rehabilitation nursing is not recommended as an entry level position. The ideal professional in the cardiac rehabilitation setting is the nurse with acute coronary care experience. The expertise of the coronary care unit nurse is essential to the rehab setting. Observing monitors, interpreting ECG changes, performing physical assessments, and being capable of handling a cardiac emergency are required skills. Extensive knowledge of cardiovascular anatomy, physiology, and pathology is equally essential.

To assure nursing effectiveness in cardiac rehabilitation, an organized approach is needed. Two primary considerations must be incorporated into rehab nursing methodology. First, the cardiac rehabilitation process is dynamic. A program adaptable to individual patients and their changing needs is essential. Second, the process is continuous from the time of diagnosis through the formal health care system and for the remainder of the patient's life. Rehab nursing approaches limited to isolated cardiac events tend to be ineffective.

In this text, the authors offer an approach to cardiac rehabilitation nursing that encompasses the features of adaptability and continuity. The model recommended for cardiac rehabilitation nursing practice is illustrated in the following figure. This model blends two already recognized systems into a functional framework.

Continuity of rehab care is provided through implementation of the "Phases" of cardiac rehabilitation as outlined by the American Heart

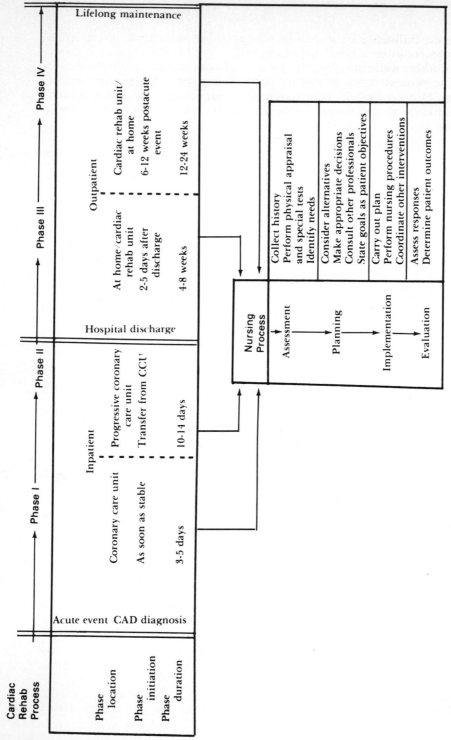

Figure I. A model for nursing practice in cardiac rehabilitation.

4

Association.[4] Individuality and adaptability are provided through use of the nursing process in each rehab phase.

The authors well realize that no definitive lines separate the components of the nursing process. We also realize that the rehab process is continuous, not segmental. However, we believe that the approach suggested here provides a nursing structure that will result in the highest quality of patient care in cardiac rehabilitation.

References

1. FRENCH, R., *The Dynamics of Health Care* (New York: McGraw-Hill Book Company, 1974), p. 1.
2. TASK FORCE ON CARDIOVASCULAR REHABILITATION, *Needs and Opportunities for Rehabilitating the Coronary Heart Disease Patient* (Bethesda, Maryland: National Heart and Lung Institute, National Institutes of Health, 1974), p. vii.
3. AMERICAN HEART ASSOCIATION, COUNCIL ON CARDIOVASCULAR NURSING, and AMERICAN NURSES' ASSOCIATION, DIVISION ON MEDICAL-SURGICAL NURSING PRACTICE, *Standards of Cardiovascular Nursing Practice* (Kansas City: American Nurses' Association, 1975).
4. WENGER, N. K., *Coronary Care, Rehabilitation After Myocardial Infarction* (New York: American Heart Association, 1973).

unit 1

phase I cardiac rehabilitation

1

background and basics of phase I cardiac rehabilitation

Behavioral Objectives

After completion of this chapter, the reader should be able to:

- cite two events which illustrate progress in management of cardiac disease in recent years.
- state the purpose of a Phase I cardiac rehab program.
- name at least six categories of nursing knowledge and six nursing skills required for nursing practice in a cardiac rehab setting.
- discuss three essential attitudes characteristic of a practitioner in cardiac rehab.
- identify a useful approach for preparing a job description for cardiac rehab nursing.
- list at least five complications of bed rest and explain the underlying physiology of each.
- present three facts in support of using a bedside commode in place of a bedpan.
- name in sequence the three psychological states the patient usually experiences during a coronary care unit (CCU) stay.

Introduction

Two statistical items dramatize progress made during the last two decades in handling the epidemic of cardiac disease. First, in the 1970s mortality rates from cardiac disease began to decline. The total number of cardiovascular deaths in 1975 fell below one million.[1] The reason for the changing trend has not been isolated, but it can be assumed that intensified efforts in public education about risk factor modification and early recognition of heart attack symptoms, coupled with generally improving health consciousness, played a major role.

The second statistic of significance which obviously contributes to the decreased mortality is the increase in inhospital survivors of acute myocardial infarction (MI), directly attributable to coronary care units. In the early 1960s, a mortality rate of 30 to 35 percent was anticipated in patients with a myocardial infarction admitted to a hospital. With the evolution of the CCU, the death rate has dropped to 10 to 20 percent.[2-5]

Originally conceived to provide specialized emergency care in the event of cardiac arrest, cardiac units soon refocused their attention on crisis prevention through dysrhythmia detection. In the 1970s, the CCU matured with the capability of early recognition and sophisticated handling of any number of potentially life-threatening cardiac complications.

As the specialty has evolved, so too has the specialist. The CCU nurse of the 1970s is not just a "rhythm watcher" as was her predecessor of the 1960s; she is a highly skilled professional capable of assessing cardiac patients for any complication that could arise and of providing the critical nursing care that is needed. Whereas critical care nurses of today receive formal education, as well as guided bedside experience, early CCU nurses usually relied on on-the-job training, self-study, and an occasional physician lecture.

Table 1-1 presents a comparison of typical CCU nursing responsibilities then and now.

Table 1-1
CCU Nursing: Then and Now

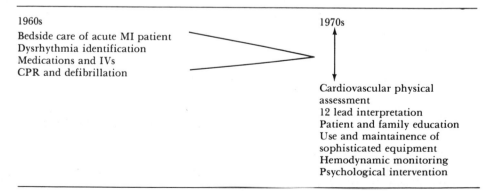

1960s

Bedside care of acute MI patient
Dysrhythmia identification
Medications and IVs
CPR and defibrillation

1970s

Cardiovascular physical assessment
12 lead interpretation
Patient and family education
Use and maintainence of sophisticated equipment
Hemodynamic monitoring
Psychological intervention

The units themselves have changed. Originally, acute cardiac units were designed to provide *complete* rest for the patient. Physically, patients rested, but the psychological stresses of being completely severed from the outside real world were profound. To some patients, the CCU was like a prison to which they vowed never to return (and, it is hoped, they haven't).

Visitors were usually discouraged by being permitted only token visits of 15 to 20 minutes three or four times a day. The patients were not even permitted cold water to drink because of the believed danger of dysrhythmia provocation!

Today, the theme of most CCUs and combination critical care units is that of optimal physical and psychological patient care. Daily orientation to the outside world is provided by use of clocks, calendars, radios, televisions, newspapers, and picture windows. Visiting hours are liberal, helping to allay both patient and family fears and frustrations. The bedside commode has replaced the bedpan as more natural and less energy demanding. And most patients are able to enjoy the luxuries of feeding themselves, drinking ice water[6], and opening their own mail. These CCU developments have each played a part in reducing cardiac catastrophes.

As briefly reviewed here, primary prevention and critical care efforts have provided an increasing number of cardiac survivors. It remains for cardiac rehabilitation efforts to transport the patient from the point of survival to the state of health.

Purpose

As stated in the Preface and evidenced in the Contents, each text unit corresponds to a phase of the cardiac rehabilitation process described in the introductory chapter. Chapters within each unit follow a recurring pattern corresponding to the sequence of the nursing process with the addition of the first chapter to each unit entitled "Background and Basics."

The practice of nursing according to the four-step process of assessment, planning, implementation, and evaluation borrows its logic from the scientific method.[7] The value of the process approach can be seen in the form, direction, and control it has given to the patient care provided by the largest health care profession.

Application of the nursing process in any area of health care cannot begin without scientific information—information about the "whys" and "wherefores" of the nursing challenge at hand. Therefore, the purpose of the background chapter beginning each unit is to provide background information and basic nursing insight as to what kind of nursing care is needed in each cardiac rehab phase and why.

Throughout the text, the nursing process approach is used from two viewpoints. First and most specifically, the process is described as it is applied to patient care in cardiac rehab. Next and often simultaneously, the logic and sequence of the process concept are applied to the rehab program as an entity in itself. The resulting material is a combination of practical patient care and realistic program organization.

Phase I Cardiac Rehabilitation

Phase I, the overture of a comprehensive cardiac rehabilitation program, begins at the time a diagnosis of cardiac disease is made. Commencement is subtle with such simple nursing actions as explaining the patient's strange environment. The purpose of a Phase I program is to reduce the physical and psychological complications that frequently accompany an acute myocardial infarction.

Nursing Requisites for Cardiac Rehab Practice

As a nursing specialty, successful cardiac rehabilitation practice requires a specific knowledge base, selected skills, and an attitude appropriate to long-term care. Major nursing requirements are listed in Table 1-2. The cognitive requirements, the things a nurse needs to know, and the psychomotor requirements, the things a nurse should be able to do, are generally met by nurses with specialty training and experience in coronary and/or critical care.

Table 1-2
Background Requirements for Cardiac Rehabilitation Nursing Practice

Cognitive Requisites	Psychomotor Requisites	Affective Requisites
Knowledge base to include	Skills to perform	Attitude that reflects
Cardiac anatomy	Cardiovascular physical	Assertiveness
Cardiovascular physiology	assessments	
Pathophysiology of	Inspection	
Coronary artery disease	Palpation	
Myocardial infarction	Percussion	
Risk factors	Auscultation	
Cardiovascular physical	Emergency cardiac care	Optimism
assessments	Defibrillation	
Rationale	Intravenous fluids	
Normal/abnormal	Medications	
Electrocardiography	Cardiopulmonary	
Normal ECG	resuscitation	
Dysrhythmia identification	ECG assessments	Leadership
12 lead interpretation	Monitoring techniques	
Emergency cardiac care	12 lead ECG recording	
Communication concepts		
Psychosocial awareness		

Affective requirements listed deserve specific consideration. Assertiveness is best defined as "behavior which enables a person to act in his/her own best interests, to stand up for himself/herself without undue anxiety, to express his/her honest feelings comfortably, or to exercise his/her own rights without denying the rights of others."[8] As the voice of a new cardiac rehab program and as the ombudsman for each of its patients, the nurse must be willing and able to effectively communicate the needs of her program, express the rights of her patients, and make recommendations for health care progress. Cardiac rehab nursing is not for the timid and shy, or for the impulsive and flamboyant.

A positive outlook is needed in any new health care program where initial inroads may be few and obstacles many. Optimism can be contagious to other personnel and patients alike. Cardiac rehab nursing is not for the easily depressed, or for chronic carriers of gloom.

Many nursing positions require leadership ability. In cardiac rehab, leadership is essential in several dimensions. First, the cardiac rehab nurse specialist must be a leader as a professional—an agent of change in a specialty where few nurse experts precede her. Second, she must be a leader as a manager— a coordinator of people from vulnerable patients to pressured physicians, of products from paper clips to computerized monitors, and of paper from appointment cards to policy manuals as large as dictionaries. Third, and sometimes most difficult, the nurse specialist in cardiac rehab practice must be a leader as a model of health. Cardiac rehab nursing is not for the lethargic overweight smoker.

Phase I Specifics

Given the general background required for cardiac rehabilitation nursing as just described, each rehab phase additionally requires certain knowledge and skills for the nursing functions inherent in the respective phase. Therefore, the cognitive and psychomotor requisites listed in each unit's background chapter are in addition to the specialty requirements shown in Table 1-2. The need for maintaining the basic attitudes previously discussed remains the same throughout the cardiac rehab continuum, so the effective listing is not repeated in the separate tables.

Phase I nursing requisites are summarized in Table 1-3. Related functions are detailed in succeeding chapters. Responsibility for Phase I rehab may belong to the CCU nurse, the cardiac rehab nurse specialist, the primary care nurse, or it may be shared.

Table 1-3
Specialized Nursing Requirements for Phase I Cardiac Rehabilitation

Cognitive	Psychomotor
Negative effects of bed rest	Operation of bedside monitoring equipment
Psychological effects of acute MI	
Appropriate early activities	
Guidelines for managing early activity	
Contraindications	
Response parameters	

Table 1-4

Job Description Outling for Cardiac Rehabilitation Nursing

Dependent Functions

Physician's Orders
Diagnostic procedures
  ECGs, lab studies
  Ambulatory monitoring
  Exercise stress testing
Therapeutic procedures
  Medications
  Dietary changes
  Exercise prescriptions

Program Policies
General institutional guidelines
under which nursing functions
are carried out may limit or
expand discretionary functions

Discretionary Functions

	Collaborative		Independent
	Physician	*Other Team Members*	
Assessment	*Patient* Admission interview		Nursing history Cardiovascular examination
	Exercise readiness	Problem identification →	
Planning	Set goals	Discuss options →	Consider available alternatives Document objectives
	Make choices		
Implementation		Carry out plan →	
Evaluation	Transfer discharge interview	Review program effectiveness Disposition and follow-up	Assess change and adjust plan Document progress Measure and document patient outcomes

Job Description

A question that seems to arise naturally from any consideration of position requirements is that of "job descriptions." What are the responsibilities and functions of cardiac rehab nurses? The answer can be found between the covers of this book. To rephrase the philosophy expressed in the introductory chapter: the role of the nurse in cardiac rehabilitation is to utilize the nursing process to fulfill the goal stated in the definition of cardiac rehabilitation—optimal health for cardiac patients.

Written job descriptions for cardiac rehab nursing can be organized in a variety of formats depending upon institutional policies and related nursing philosophies. Table 1-4 provides a general job description useful for cardiac rehab nursing as presented in this text.

The format recommended is based on the following rationale:

- Nursing functions can be divided into dependent and discretionary.
- Dependent functions can be subdivided into two categories:
  absolute—in the sense that the nurse has no control over the decision dictating the function (physician's orders).
  relative—in the sense that the nurse may have input in defining the function, but not necessarily in the final decision (program policies).
- Discretionary functions describe functions performed in the nursing process and can be subdivided into two categories:
  independent—those functions the nurse is able to carry out unaided.
  collaborative—those functions enhanced by participation of other rehab team members.
  Depending upon the patient, the circumstances, the resources, and so on, the nurse decides whether singular or group effort can best accomplish the goal at hand, thus the term "discretionary."

Use of this job description approach allows for expansion by detailing specific functions and tasks appropriate to the exact position being described under the general categories.

Bases of Phase I Cardiac Rehabilitation

Physiological Basis

Bed rest, the classic treatment for acute myocardial infarction has accrued a host of well-defined complications, some equally as serious as the problem for which the treatment was instituted. Deconditioning, the collective term commonly used to describe the deleterious effects of bed rest, can be countered by early mobilization of the stabilized myocardial infarction patient. Problems resulting from bed rest include the following.

Muscular Weakness. Distressing to the cardiac patient, the decrease in contractile strength of body musculature which occurs with bed rest tends to reinforce his fears that perhaps he is more seriously ill than he has been told. Generalized weakness increases the muscular demand for oxygen when activity is attempted and indirectly places an added strain on the heart.

Tachycardia. As deconditioning increases, the heart rate required to perform a given activity will increase in response to the additional muscular need for oxygen.[9-10] As the heart rate increases, shortening the diastolic-filling time, the danger of further myocardial ischemia increases. The faster the heart beats, the more oxygen the myocardium requires. Sufficient delivery depends, in part, upon the condition of the coronary circulation.

Thrombus Formation. Thrombus formation in the lower extremities is another complication of bed rest. The incidence of thrombus formation appears to be directly proportional to the number of days the patient remains in bed.[11] This may be due to the decrease in circulating blood volume, with a greater decrease in plasma volume than in red blood cell mass, increasing the viscosity of the blood.[12] Probably, the decrease in extremity movement and muscular contractions which ordinarily promote venous return predisposes to this condition. The ultimate danger of prolonged venostasis is pulmonary embolism.

Orthostatic Hypotension. A frequent experience of the patient who has been on bed rest for a few days, orthostatic hypotension is the result of gradual loss of vasomotor responsiveness. As the patient assumes an upright position, the blood tends to pool in the lower extremities, decreasing circulating blood volume, venous return, and cardiac output. As the blood pressure drops, the patient feels dizzy, shaky, and faint.[13-14]

Pulmonary Problems. Effects of bed rest on pulmonary function are of particular importance to the cardiac patient. A decrease in lung volume and vital capacity may predispose to atelectasis and secretion accumulation.[15-16] The increase in pulmonary blood volume which occurs in the supine position may lead to increased pulmonary congestion in patients with compromised left ventricular function.

Blood Chemistry Changes. Additional complications include a decrease in serum protein concentrations and a negative nitrogen and calcium balance. These factors may influence the healing process and myocardial electrical stability during healing.

Valsalva Effects. The patient who is on bed rest performs the Valsalva maneuver frequently throughout the day as he attempts to reposition himself in bed. The physiological changes that result from this breath-holding action can be threatening to an already weakened ischemic cardiac muscle. Figure 1-1 illustrates the sequence of Valsalva-produced responses. It has been estimated that patients on bed rest use the Valsalva maneuver 10 to 20 times per hour.[17]

Constipation. While not as immediately life-threatening as other complications of bed rest, constipation is a frequent result of bed rest, causing patient discomfort.

The generalized decrease in activity and lowered metabolism associated with bed rest may predispose to constipation. Further, the use of a bedpan places the patient in an unnatural position for defecation which interferes with normal reflexes and mechanisms, increasing the likelihood of use of the abdominal muscles and the Valsalva maneuver to effect bowel movement. It is not only unnatural and uncomfortable to have to use a bedpan, but it is embarrassing as

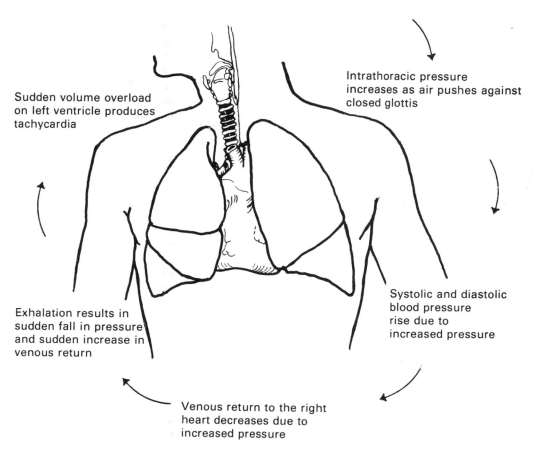

Valsalva initiated by
breath holding with
immobilization of chest muscles

Intrathoracic pressure
increases as air pushes against
closed glottis

Sudden volume overload
on left ventricle produces
tachycardia

Systolic and diastolic
blood pressure
rise due to
increased pressure

Exhalation results in
sudden fall in pressure
and sudden increase in
venous return

Venous return to the right
heart decreases due to
increased pressure

Figure 1-1.   Effects of a valsalva maneuver.

well. Due to embarrassment, the patient may deny any urge to defecate as long as possible, compounding the problem of constipation.

The metabolic requirements of using a bedpan and using the bedside commode have both been calculated. It has been found that it requires about four times the resting energy level to use a bedpan as compared to about three times the resting energy level to use the bedside commode.[18] In view of this, as well as the unnatural position of the bedpan and the embarrassment, it would appear that use of the bedside commode is by far the better choice.

Psychological Basis

Given the experience of having a heart attack, being admitted to an intensive care unit, suffering pain and discomfort, being isolated from family, awakening in a foreign environment with strange equipment—is it any wonder that cardiac patients experience anxiety? Given the realization that one's heart has been damaged, and all the possible effects this may have on his life and the lives of those he loves—is it any wonder that depression is a common characteristic following myocardial infarction?

Patients react to the stress of acute myocardial infarction in their own individual manner or style. Reaction is dependent upon their perception of the problem and their customary methods of coping with serious problems. They may evoke various defense mechanisms and coping behaviors. If they are successful in dealing with this insult, a sense of hopefulness about their life will be maintained.

In a study by Hackett and Cassem, anxiety experienced by patients usually stemmed either from fear of sudden death or from the appearance of symptoms, such as breathlessness, chest pain, or complications. Another symptom which evoked anxiety was the sensation of weakness.[19] The degree of anxiety was unrelated to the actual seriousness of the illness or to socioeconomic background.

Denial is a common defense mechanism employed by the cardiac patient, and in Hackett and Cassem's hypothetical schedule of the onset of emotional and behavioral reactions of the CCU patient, denial is at its peak during the second day. Thereafter, the predominate emotion is depression, beginning about day three.[20] These psychiatrists suggest that all myocardial infarction patients be treated for depression ". . . best accomplished by a rehabilitation program that begins no later than the depression begins, namely on or before the third CCU day."[21]

References

1. STAMLER, J., et al., "Introduction to Risk Factors in Coronary Artery Disease," *Heart and Lung,* January-February 1978, p. 131.
2. VOORMAN, D., "Critical-Care Nursing: Reflections and Forecasts," *Heart and Lung,* May-June 1976, p. 361.
3. MELTZER, L., et al., *Concepts and Practices of Intensive Care Nurse Specialists* (Bowie, Maryland: Charles Press, 1969), p. 50.
4. O'BRIEN, M. R., FLOOD, M., and GRACE, W. J., "Coronary Care 1977," *Cardio-Vascular Nursing* (New York: American Heart Association, January-February 1977), pp. 1-6.
5. PINNEO, R., "Nursing in a Coronary Care Unit," *Cardio-Vascular Nursing* (New York: American Heart Association, January-February 1967), pp. 1-4.
6. HOUSER, D., "Ice Water for MI Patients? Why Not? *American Journal of Nursing,* March 1976, p. 432.
7. GANONG, J. M. and GANONG, W. L., *Nursing Management* (Germantown, Maryland: Aspen Systems Corporation, 1976), pp. 19-25.

8. ALBERTI, R. E. and EMMONS, M. L., *Your Perfect Right, A Guide To Assertive Behavior,* 2nd ed. (San Luis Obispo, California: Impact Publishing Company, 1974), p. 2.

9. SALTIN, B., et al., "Response to Exercise After Bed Rest and After Training," *Circulation,* November 1968, pp. 1-78.

10. CARDUS, D., "Effects of 10 Days Recumbency on Response to the Bicycle Ergometer Test," *Aerospace Medicine,* 1969, pp. 933-999.

11. OLSON, E. V., "The Hazards of Immobility," *American Journal of Nursing,* April 1967, pp. 780-797.

12. COMMITTEE ON EXERCISE, *Exercise Testing and Training of Individuals with Heart Disease or at High Risk for Its Development: A Handbook for Physicians* (New York: American Heart Association, 1975), pp. 20-21.

13. OLSON, *op. cit.,* pp. 780-797.

14. COMMITTEE ON EXERCISE, *op. cit.,* pp. 20-21.

15. OLSON, *op. cit.,* pp. 780-797.

16. COMMITTEE ON EXERCISE, *op. cit.,* pp. 20-21.

17. OLSON, *op. cit.,* pp. 780-797.

18. CARDIAC RECONDITIONING and WORK EVALUATION UNIT, *Exercise Equivalents* (Denver, Colorado: Colorado Heart Association, 1970). p. 12.

19. HACKETT, T. P. and CASSEM, N. H., *Coronary Care: Patient Psychology* (New York: American Heart Association, 1975), pp. 1-15.

20. *Ibid.,* pp. 10-11.

21. CASSEM, N. H. and HACKETT, T. P., "Psychological Rehabilitation of Myocardial Infarction Patients in the Acute Phase," *Heart and Lung,* May-June 1973, pp. 382-387.

2

assessments for phase I cardiac rehabilitation

Behavioral Objectives

After completion of this chapter, the reader should be able to:
- define "assessment" and discuss its significance in the nursing process.
- differentiate patient "needs" from patient "problems."
- describe a useful classification system for patient needs and problems in cardiac rehab practice and discuss its theoretical base.
- relate the importance of self-assessment in cardiac rehab nursing.
- discuss how to assess a patient's readiness to learn.

Introduction

Assessment, the first step in the nursing process, may be defined as the collection and analysis of information about the patient's health status.[1] Composed of both subjective information, that which is supplied by the patient, and objective data, results from tests and measurements on the patient, thorough assessment is essential to cardiac rehab nursing practice. The collection segment of assessment requires specialized technical and mental cognitive skills. Once gathered, data are analyzed and their significance determined. Correct analysis depends upon current, comprehensive nursing knowledge.

Nursing Assessments in Cardiac Rehabilitation: An Overview

The cardiac rehabilitation process is continuous from the time of diagnosis through lifelong maintenance. However, as the patient progresses into each phase in the sequence, thorough assessment is required to determine the patient's health status at that point. If the nurse specialist assumes responsibility for the patient's health care during the particular rehab phase being entered, she is also responsible for carrying out an investigation to determine the foundation upon which rehab care will be built.

Initial Assessments in Each Rehab Phase

The purpose of the second chapter in each unit is to identify nursing assessments specific to each rehab phase. The complexity of these initial determinations varies from phase to phase, but at the very least, initiation of each phase involves review of the patient's health history and progress to date and a condensed physical examination. Even in cases in which the same nurse follows the patient throughout rehabilitation, assessments described for each phase are completed to update the nurse's awareness and assure that health planning is based on the most current patient information.

Classification of Health Problems

Once assessment procedures have been completed and data obtained are documented, the nurse is next responsible for sifting and sorting the information and extracting from it health concerns that require nursing intervention. Nursing conclusions drawn from the assessment analysis, also known as nursing diagnoses, must be organized in a way that will be conducive to planning and implementing nursing care.

A number of methods have been described for classifying assessment findings. The approach suggested here is practical in its organization and can be realistically applied in cardiac rehab nursing. Maslow's theory provides the classification basis.

According to Maslow, human behavior is the result of striving to fulfill intrinsic "needs." These needs occur in an ascending order of importance, or hierarchy. The level at which a person is operating at a given time depends upon the dominant need at that time. As each need in the scale is met, a person progresses to the next higher need. When problems arise, upward progression is halted or regression to lower needs may occur. The following is a summary of Maslow's hierarchy:

Physiological needs—needs for life and health; all physical functions can be considered here.
Safety needs—needs for stability, security, and freedom from threat and danger.
Social needs—needs for satisfactory relationships and acceptance by others.
Ego needs—needs for recognition, status, and accomplishment.
Self-actualization needs—needs for independence, creativity, and use of personal potential.[2-6]

With this theory in mind, the term needs is used to mean expected influences on behavior. As such, many needs can be anticipated throughout the rehab process and assistance toward their fulfillment planned in advance. On the other hand, "problems" can be considered abnormal conditions or circumstances that interfere with need fulfillment.

Problem-solving begins with problem identification through nursing assessments. Grouping problems into categories of health concern correlated to the need hierarchy simplifies use of the concepts just described and eases application of theory to practice (see Figure 2-1). Assessment concludes with the patient's problems being reorganized as physiological, psychosocial, or educational.

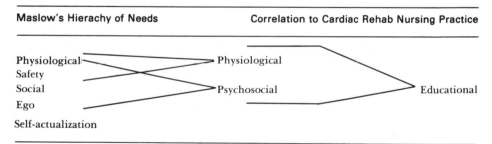

Figure 2-1.   Suggested classification system for cardiac rehab nursing.

Self-assessment

As discussed thus far, assessment has been an externally applied science. But in cardiac rehab nursing, as in other health care settings requiring long-term, intense contact with patients and families, the cornerstone to nursing effectiveness is self-awareness. Assessment of personal and professional self, therefore, should be a standard part of a nurse's commitment to begin or continue cardiac rehabilitation practice.

General attitudes desirable for cardiac rehab practice were discussed in Chapter 1. Introspection can identify the presence or absence of characteristics that compose attitudes. Self-analysis can begin with the following questions:

Do I project a positive outlook?

Do I project a high degree of self-esteem?

Am I consistent in my interactions with people?

Am I trustworthy?

Am I consistent in health teaching?

Do I kindle enthusiasm about what I am teaching?

Do I refrain from discussing personal problems, departmental problems, and the problems of other patients?

Do I truly respect patients as people with their own rights, or do I see them as just another "cardiac?"

Do I respect the beliefs of others or try to impose mine?

Am I nonjudgmental, or do I judge others according to my own value system?

What are my prejudices?

What do my mode of dress, personal hygiene, posture, gestures, tone of voice, attentiveness (or lack of it) project to patients?

Do I practice what I preach or do my habits display what I ask my patients to discard?

Am I willing to constantly strive to update my knowledge and techniques in a rapidly developing field?

Certain nursing roles incorporated in cardiac rehab practice may require an even greater depth of self-understanding. The role of patient advocate requires empathy. Being cognizant of patients's emotions helps foster creativity and increases the likelihood that rehab needs will be met in the way most meaningful to the patient.

How can a healthy nurse really know what it's like to be a cardiac patient? A few "empathy exercises" may help. For example, when lying in bed unable to sleep, imagine that you have suffered a heart attack and are in CCU. Seriously consider the impact this unexpected event is having on your life, your habits, your future plans, and your loved ones. This role-playing may not help you sleep better, but it may help you become a better cardiac rehab nurse. Another example, put yourself and your family on the low-fat, low-calorie diet prescribed for most of your patients. Learn firsthand the problems of food shopping, cooking, and adherence accompanying this behavior change.

The role of sex counselor is threatening to many nurses. Yet sexuality is intrinsic to being human. Victorian attitudes often inhibit discussion of the influence heart disease may have on continuation or resumption of sexual activity even when such concerns are voiced by the patient.

The nurse who plans to meet the need for counseling patients on safely enjoying the powerful and purposeful human sexual response must be comfortable with her own sexuality.[7] Personal insight will increase as knowledge of human sexuality expands. The cardiac rehab nurse should avail herself of learning experiences related to sexual understanding. Knowledge about human sexuality and good communication skills are the bases for dealing with the sexual concerns of patients and their significant others.

The role of nurse educator is a complex one requiring extensive knowledge of the subjects to be taught, good teaching skills, and an attitude that will stimulate learning. Good nurse educators in cardiac rehab are not born; they are developed over time. Their knowledge is correct and current. They know which teaching techniques apply when. They know their limitations and weaknesses and are constantly striving to improve.

As discussed throughout this text, results of teaching can be measured and effectiveness objectively determined. Frequently, self-assessment by the nurse educator is of added value. Although nurse educators seldom think of themselves as sales agents, their role does have similarities to that of the salesperson. A sales analogy provides a stimulating example of self-assessment. Consider that you are trying to "sell" an educational topic to a doubtful patient-buyer:

- A salesperson entices prospective buyers to purchase an item because of the benefits they will get from owning it; the educator must have the ability to identify patients' needs and create within the patient the desire to have that need satisfied.
- A consumer will buy more readily from a salesperson who can give a clear understanding of the product's use; the educator must have a firm understanding of her "product." The patient will accept clear, concise, factual information much more readily than vagueness or inaccuracy.
- Salespeople with indifferent attitudes seldom achieve "Salesperson of the Year"; educators must be able to project enthusiasm about their "product."
- Sales without service is less attractive than a product with a service warranty; educators need to offer maintenance service; that is, there should be a plan whereby the patient has access to support, reassurance, and assistance in adjusting and maintaining life-style changes important to his health. The cardiac rehab continuum provides such ongoing service.

Phase I Assessments

Many nursing assessments are carried out in the CCU. Those most obvious are the sophisticated measurements necessary for good nursing and medical management during the acute stage. Between the specialized techniques, and no less dramatic to total health care, are the Phase I rehab-related assessments.

Educational Readiness

Patient education should begin as the patient enters the CCU. Much of the education performed in this very early stage is directed toward allaying fears, reducing anxieties, and helping the patient accept his diagnosis and treatment plan. Here the groundwork is laid for more in-depth teaching and the active involvement of the patient in setting objectives and goals for himself during his progression through later rehab phases.

After the diagnosis is made, information concerning what a heart attack is and how the injury heals may be offered briefly. Readiness to learn about the heart attack and its treatment is closely tied to the psychological state of the patient. Some patients in the early stage of recovery simply do not want to hear they have had a heart attack, and they will not remember information offered them. Others may only want to hear certain things and no more. The nurse must be able to recognize the patient's needs and offer that information which he is ready to receive. She must also be prepared to repeat the information and/or expand it at a future time, because patients in Phase I frequently remember very little that is told to them.

Part of the process of identifying the patient's early educational needs involves eliciting information the patient already has regarding his condition. Often, patients have misinformation which keeps their anxiety level so high that they are unable to cope with the diagnosis or treatment plan and, thus, educational advancement is hindered.

Ask the patient what he knows about a heart attack, why it happens, how it affects the heart, what the healing process is like. Evaluate his level of understanding, reinforce his correct information and correct his misconceptions. This need not be done in a formal teaching period during this phase, but could best be accomplished by conversation during routine nursing care.

The nurse should be a good listener, staying alert for clues that the patient gives indicating a desire for information that may help him accept his diagnosis or treatment plan. Talking with the nurse may allow the patient to view his circumstances more realistically and, thus, develop coping mechanisms to reduce his anxieties. Sometimes, the best service the nurse can give the patient in this regard is to allow him to ventilate and sort his own feelings. Support, encouragement, and information can be provided as requested.

If the patient is given an understanding of his condition in a way that is not frightening, he may be able to accept the diagnosis more easily. If he is not given an adequate explanation or does not have a good understanding, he is likely to imagine the worst. Pictures of a healthy heart, of an infarcted heart, and of a healed heart with scar tissue evident are good teaching aids to have readily available in the CCU.

Patients who are actively denying their diagnosis pose a problem which is not easily solved. It is likely that denial, an important coping mechanism, is necessary to the patient's emotional well-being. It should not be reinforced by the staff nor should it be destroyed. This coping mechanism may be necessary for the patient because of erroneous information about the disease or recovery process, and such a possibility should be investigated prior to teaching. The patient who continues to deny will not internalize what is taught. That is, he will be unable to personally accept that what is being taught pertains to him.

The patient's actions frequently indicate the need for teaching. Consider, for example, the patient who strains and stretches to pull himself up in bed. He obviously needs to understand the effects such struggling may have on his heart and should be told the proper action to take if he feels he needs to be up higher in his bed. This may lead to a brief explanation of beneficial activities for cardiac patients.

Many of the patient's educational needs can be anticipated, and although it may not be appropriate to go into detail during Phase I, simple explanations should be given. Discussions initiated here can be expanded later in the rehab process when the patient is more receptive to teaching. For example, activity restrictions: Straining your muscles causes extra work for your heart. Most tasks can be performed in a manner that will allow you to do things for yourself, yet provide the rest your heart requires. (Followed by demonstration of shaving or hair combing with elbows resting on overbed table.) Medications: This pill helps you relax and get the rest you need. Your heart doesn't have to work as hard when you are relaxed, so it is not only helping you be a little more content while in the unit, but it is helping give your heart a chance to heal. Later, when you feel more up to it, we will discuss your medications in detail so you have a good understanding of them.

Such simple initial explanations can be offered regarding diet, other medications, the importance of alerting the staff to any symptoms experienced, and proper methods of performing activities.

Almost every contact the nurse has with the patient in routine care offers an opportunity for education, support, reassurance, or clarification of a point. The patient's learning needs cannot always be anticipated. The nurse should be prepared with an understanding of the patient's condition and treatment plan, and a thorough knowledge of the disease process and its sequelae in order to be able to give information which is factual and pertinent whenever requested.

Physiological Stability

Rehab activities in the CCU are best initiated at the earliest possible time consistent with patient safety. This may mean that the patient will begin prescribed activities as soon as the day after admission if he is physiologically stable. Assessment of stability includes review of the patient's heart rate and rhythm, blood pressure, serial ECGs, lab studies, and cardiovascular examination findings. The acute myocardial infarction patient who is free from pain and does not display signs of cardiac failure or dysrhythmias will benefit from activities designed to prevent deconditioning when these are performed within his physiological capabilities.[8-12]

Summary: Sample Case

Each chapter in this text (with the exception of the background chapters) concludes with excerpts from a patient case illustrative of the concepts and functions discussed in the preceding pages. The case utilized is continuous through successive chapters demonstrating both intraphase and interphase relationships in cardiac rehabilitation nursing care.

In order to highlight cardiac rehabilitation, only support data relative to rehab are reproduced. It should be understood, particularly with the inpatient excerpts, that other medical and nursing care occurred simultaneously. To emphasize planning, initial "rehab care plans" are presented for each phase. It should be understood that the plan is changed as the patient progresses.

(Patient ID Stamp)

<table>
<tr><td>C. P.</td><td>ADMISSION
HISTORY</td></tr>
</table>

5/1/XX - 10 a.m.

42-year-old, white, male, school teacher, owns and works a farm, admitted to CCU via ER for earlier chest pain.

CHIEF COMPLAINT: One episode of chest tightness.

HISTORY OF PRESENT ILLNESS: While feeding his cattle this morning, developed a heavy feeling or tightness in his anterior superior chest. Radiated to both sides of his neck and to his right arm. The pain was not associated with deep breathing and did not have a pleuritic type catch on respirations.

The pain was worse with exertion and caused him to walk slowly to his home and lie in bed. After lying in bed for some time, the pain subsided and has not recurred. He denies SOB, nausea, vomiting, or diaphoresis with this pain but did feel cold. Pain lasted approximately 2 hours.

PAST MEDICAL HISTORY: Had a similar episode of tightness in his jaws 8 years ago. ECG at that time was normal and apparently, according to family physician, ECG has not changed since then. Chest pain has not given him any problems in the past 8 years.

He was admitted to this hospital approximately 12 years ago for viral encephalitis. He stated he had childhood diseases but denies rheumatic fever, scarlet fever, TB, pneumonia. He has had a history of kidney infection. Denies any other systems diseases. Denies allergies. No medicines.

FAMILY HISTORY: Father is alive at 74. CVA and being treated for hypertension. Mother is 69 with hypertension. Had a brother who died in this hospital in 1974 at age 45 with MI. Another brother age 36 with hypertension and a third brother age 33 alive and healthy. One sister alive and healthy. Denies FH of cancer, TB, diabetes mellitus, or blood dyscrasias. Denies smoking or alcohol use.

REVIEW OF SYSTEMS: Denies any tremors, weight change, night sweats, fever. Skin—denies any changes. Head—frontal headaches usually occurring about 3 in the afternoon and usually relieved by aspirin. Denies syncope, Eyes—noticed some blurring lately but feels he needs new glasses, denies photophobia. Ears—denies discharges, does have some ringing and buzzing in his ears on occasions, has been present for some time. Denies any dizziness. Nose—denies any epistaxsis or sinusitis. Throat—denies hoarseness, redness, or dysphasia. Respiratory—denies hemoptysis, sputum, or dyspnea. Muscles—without complaints. Cardiovascular—per chief complaint but denies palpitation, tachycardia, or vertigo. GI without complaints. GU without complaints. Neuro—states that he is a nervous individual.

_J. D._ , M.D.

(Patient ID Stamp)		
	C. P.	**ADMISSION** **EXAMINATION**

(Summary of Physical Examination and Lab Studies)

5/1/XX

PHYSICAL EXAMINATION: Well-developed, well-nourished male, no acute distress at present. B/P 148/98, P 98. No other pertinent physical findings.

LAB STUDIES: CPK ↑ 225. Other enzymes normal on admission. CBC, urinalysis, SMA 6 and 12—normal. Triglycerides 106, protein electrophoresis normal. Cholesterol on admission 255. Chest x-ray and cardiac series normal. Admission ECG: ST ↑ II, III, AVF.

IMPRESSION: Acute inferior MI.

_J.D._ M.D.

(Patient ID Stamp)		
	C. P.	**CARDIAC REHAB PROGRESS NOTES**

Date/Time	PROGRESS NOTES
5/1/XX 2 p.m.	42-year-old male patient, married, daughter age 9, son age 6 admitted earlier
	today. Stopped in to introduce myself and review admission findings. Admission
	assessment:
	S. Short discussion with patient. Revealed his brother died 2 years ago from
	AMI, "now it's my turn." Appears very anxious visibly nervous and shaky.
	Concerned about his farm, "what happens now? There's no one else to look
	after the farm."
	O. Reviewed H & P, initial lab results and ECG, and rhythm strips and CCU notes
	since admission.
	A. No further acute problems. Condition stable.
	P. Questions and comments responded to briefly. Advised that full details will
	be provided once he's rested. Rehab planning initiated. Will check with Dr. J.
	D. for orders.
	$\mathcal{N.D.}$ R.N.

References

1. BOWER, F. L., *The Process of Planning Nursing Care*, 2nd ed. (St. Louis, Missouri: The C. V. Mosby Company, 1977), p. 11.
2. MASLOW, A. H., *Motivation and Personality*, 2nd ed. (New York: Harper & Row, Publishers, Inc., 1970), pp. 3-12.
3. GANONG, J. M. and GANONG, W. L., *Nursing Management* (Germantown, Maryland: Aspen Systems Corporation, 1976), pp. 323-328.
4. KRON, T., *The Management of Patient Care*, 3rd ed. (Philadelphia: W. B. Saunders Company, 1971), pp. 98-100.
5. BECKNELL, E. P. and SMITH D. M., *System of Nursing Practice* (Philadelphia: F.A. Davis Company, 1975), pp. 10-12.
6. JONES, P. S., "An Adaptation Model for Nursing Practice," *American Journal of Nursing*, November 1978, pp. 1900-1906.
7. KROZY, R., "Becoming Comfortable with Sexual Assessment,"*American Journal of Nursing*, June 1978, pp. 1036-1038.
8. BARRY, E. M., KNIGHT, S. A., and ACKER, J. E., "Hospital Program for Cardiac Rehabilitation," *American Journal of Nursing*, December 1972, pp. 2174-2177.
9. HASKELL, W. L., "Physical Activity After Myocardial Infarction," *American Journal of Cardiology*, May 20, 1974, pp. 776-783.
10. NAUGHTON, J. P., "The Contribution of Regular Physical Activity to the Ambulatory Care of Cardiac Patients," *Postgraduate Medicine*, April 1975, pp. 51-55.
11. LAWSON, M., "Progressive Coronary Care," *Heart and Lung*, March-April 1972, pp. 240-252.
12. LAVIN, M. A., "Bed Exercises for Acute Cardiac Patients," *American Journal of Nursing*, July 1973, pp. 1226-1227.

3

planning of phase I cardiac rehabilitation

Behavioral Objectives

After completion of this chapter, the reader should be able to:

■ define "planning" and discuss its significance in the nursing process.

■ describe a planning approach useful in cardiac rehab practice that begins with a general purpose and is completed by specific, well-defined objectives.

■ present a sample format for a rehab care plan.

■ identify common nursing goals of Phase I.

■ list at least four principles upon which early activity programs should be based.

■ recommend activities appropriate to Phase I and suggest a structured approach for implementation.

■ discuss the importance of basic explanations and frequent reassurance for patient and family during Phase I.

Introduction

Planning consists of setting goals, weighing alternatives, proposing interventions, and predicting outcomes.[1] Having identified the patient's problems through assessment, nursing responsibility expands to planning, the second step in the nursing process. An extensive knowledge base is needed to plan for effective cardiac rehabilitation. Although less visible than other steps in the nursing process, planning is perhaps the most complex and challenging.

Cardiac Rehabilitation Planning: An Overview

The purpose of the third chapter in each unit is to identify nursing approaches to be considered during the planning of cardiac rehab care. In the planning chapters, the rationale of prevalent approaches is discussed and nursing functions are described in detail.

Purpose, Goals and Objectives

Cardiac rehabilitation planning needs to consider both patient similarities and dissimilarities. The planning that is described in this text occurs in a three-step funnel-like sequence, each step being a progressive refinement of the overall cardiac rehab intent.

General Phase Purpose. Each rehab phase has a purpose congruent with the achievement and maintenance of optimal health for postacute cardiac patients (see background chapter of respective phases). Although health care emphasis shifts according to the purpose of each phase, the purposes of all phases are interrelated and continuous. In addition, all categories of patient needs are addressed in each phase.

Common Nursing Goals. To stereotype all postmyocardial infarction patients as having identical problems would be a regression in nursing practice. However, experience indicates that many patients have similar needs at certain times during their recovery. Anticipating these needs and planning in advance for appropriate nursing intervention to meet them will prevent many problems and allow more nursing time and energy to be directed toward unpredictable events and the unique problems presented by individual patients.

Using the need categories described in Chapter 2, goals based on patient similarities can be drafted in anticipation of needs that usually occur in that phase. Labeled "common nursing goals," these predeterminations provide a reference for organizing nursing care. All projected nursing goals will not apply to every patient. It is part of the planning function to determine which goals are appropriate, which require modification, and which do not apply to a given patient.

Specific Patient Objectives. The third step in refining a rehab plan incorporates the patient's uniqueness. Problems specific to the patient are added to appropriate common goals and both are converted into patient objectives. Behavioral objectives (described in Chapter 8) express the projected result of the patient's participation in that phase of the cardiac rehabilitation process. Two major planning functions are necessary for the completion of patient objectives.

First, alternatives for meeting the need or solving the problem must be investigated. In other words, nursing consideration must be given to the question of what solutions are available. Second, of the available alternatives, which is best for this patient? Although the first question can usually be answered by the nurse, the second requires the active involvement of the patient. Just as the patient's input was needed to identify his health problems, the necessity of involving the patient and family in selecting rehab approaches cannot be overlooked. The patient is an active member of the cardiac rehab team. The nurse provides and clarifies information and answers questions. Choices and decisions belong to the patient.

Once the patient has expressed his choice of approaches, he and the nurse further define his goals by considering when the goals should be reached and how their achievement will be reflected in the patient's behavior. The completed objectives are then expressed in the rehab care plan.

The above planning sequence is illustrated in Figure 3-1.

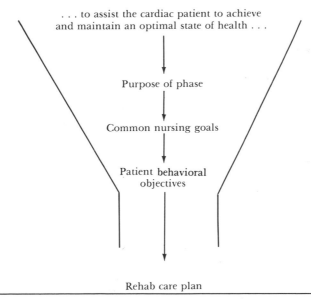

. . . to assist the cardiac patient to achieve and maintain an optimal state of health . . .

Purpose of phase

Common nursing goals

Patient behavioral objectives

Rehab care plan

Figure 3-1 Cardiac rehab planning.

The Rehab Care Plan

Formats for nursing care plans are almost as numerous as the number of health care facilities using them. Planning documentation used in the samples here is adaptable to either standard narrative charting or problem-oriented records. The term rehab care plan is used to emphasize the fact that the plan, is not solely owned by the nurse. The patient holds an equal interest. The plan represents his understanding of how to improve his health status. The nurse simply translates the patient's decisions and directions into health care language.

The rehab care plan coexists with another nursing record, the rehab progress notes (See Chapter 4), and the two should be located together in the patient's chart. The sample case summarizing Chapters 3, 8, 13, and 18 presents the initial rehab plan for respective phases.

Phase I Rehab Planning

The ultimate rehab goal of optimal health is reached one step or phase at a time. Phase I rehab points the patient in the right direction for successful recovery. Common nursing goals for Phase I cardiac rehab are shown in Table 3-1.

Table 3-1
Common Nursing Goals of Phase I Cardiac Rehabilitation

Physiological

To enable the patient to carry out routine self-care.

To prevent the negative effects of bed rest.

Psychosocial

To assist the patient and significant others in their realization of and adjustment to a sudden change in health status.

Educational

To help the patient and significant others to understand what has happened, what is being done by various health professionals, and what they can do to help themselves and each other.

Activities in CCU

Participation in self-care activities provides both the patient and family tangible and realistic assurance that the future is not as uncertain as initially imagined. Patients for whom a structured activity plan has been instituted are less likely to experience acute depression after their myocardial infarction than patients confined to prolonged bed rest. Families who observe their loved ones' ability to function on a level approaching normal are less likely to become overprotective of the patient.[2]

Activity Principles. Activity at the CCU level is designed to prevent deconditioning, while not being too stressful for the cardiovascular system. Isometric activity (See Chapter 6) and the Valsalva maneuver (See Chapter 1) should be avoided because of undesirable effects on the cardiovascular system. Promotion of self-care, maintenance of muscle tone and joint flexibility, and improvement in venous return are built into activity planning.

Several plans have been described for helping patients to progress through early rehab activities.[3-7] These and others are similarly constructed using the following principles:

- Activity should begin at low levels and progress to levels compatible with self-care functions.
- Activity should be carried out when the patient is rested; alternating activity and rest periods throughout the day is advisable.
- Activity should be meaningful and beneficial to the patient; he should understand the need for active participation in appropriate activity and purposeful avoidance of potentially harmful activity.
- Activity should be performed within the patient's individual capabilities while monitored by a knowledgeable cardiac rehab health professional.
- Activity should be explained to the patient and family to reduce anxiety and provide a sense of gradual improvement.

Activity Guidelines. As stated previously, activity should be performed within the physiological capabilities of the individual patient. Guidelines specifying acceptable and excessive responses need to be established. A sample of parameters used to guide activity is shown in Figure 3-2.

Allowable Responses	Disproportionate Responses
Heart rate Increase of 10-20 beats over resting (upper limit 120 b.p.m.)	Excessive heart rate of blood pressure change Chest pain or dyspnea Dysrhythmia or conduction disturbance
Blood pressure Increase/decrease 10-20 mm. systolic from resting	Ischemic ST segment displacement

Figure 3-2. Phase I activity guidelines. Adapted from Wenger, N. K., *Coronary Care: Rehabilitation After Myocardial Infarction* (New York: American Heart Association, 1973), p. 6; Barry, E. M., Knight, S. A., and Acker, J. E., "Hospital Program for Cardiac Rehabilitation," *American Journal of Nursing*, December 1972, pp. 2174-2177; Haskel, W. L. "Physical Activity After Myocardial Infarction," *American Journal of Cardiology*, 20 May 1974, pp. 776-783; and Amsterdam, E. A., et al., "Exercise To Put The MI Patient on His Feet," *Medical Opinion*, June 1975, pp. 12-17.

Regarding heart rate guidelines used for early activity programs, it should be emphasized that activity is not meant to escalate the patient's heart rate, but rather to keep the heart rate below a stated limit. Many patients demonstrate little or no increase in heart rate if their activity program is started early and deconditioning prevented.

Patients who are not candidates for early activity progression—those with complications such as congestive heart failure, dysrhythmias, or chest pain— may still be capable of and benefit from passive range-of-motion and deep-breathing exercises.

Activity Levels. Steps or levels of activity that most myocardial infarction patients are able to achieve while in CCU range from passive range-of-motion exercises to walking a few steps around the bed and/or sitting in a chair at the bedside. Self-care activities usually allowed include feeding, shaving, putting on makeup, brushing teeth, and washing the face, upper anterior part of the body, and genital area. Figure 3-3 illustrates a progressive plan of activity.

In addition to what activities to plan in Phase I, nursing consideration must be given to how the activities will be performed.

Activities Performed with the Arms. Eating, shaving, putting on makeup, brushing teeth, and washing are all allowable Phase I arm activities. To keep energy needs when performing these activities low, the nurse should be certain that all items needed by the patient are within easy reach and are ready to use. For example, food should be bite sized, liquids should be poured, lids removed, and so on.

Instructions regarding arm activities should include the following:

- Rest elbows as much as possible when performing the task, by either placing the elbows on pillow supports or resting them on the overbed table.
- Use forearm, wrist, hand, and head movements to perform such tasks as self-feeding, shaving, brushing the teeth, and so on. It is usually not necessary to involve shoulder motion or hold the arms at shoulder level in these types of activities.
- Try to reduce arm tension as much as possible. Do not wring the washcloth or scrub vigorously. Do not try to tie or untie the gown behind the back. Do not hold the arms overhead to style hair (if the patient has more than a simple hair style, he/she will probably require assistance).
- If an activity increases fatigue or causes symptoms, inform the nurse immediately.

Activities Performed with the Legs. Initially, movements of the legs, feet, ankles knees, and hip joints may be performed by the nurse with the patient relaxed. This passive range of motion is easily carried out during a bed bath or other physical care. [12] The stable patient is likely to tolerate active manipulation of his lower extremities, that is, performance of range-of-motion exercises without the assistance of the nurse. The purpose of range-of-motion exercises is to maintain joint mobility and prevent venous stasis and muscle deconditioning.

Patients can become active participants in their recovery plan by being encouraged to perform lower extremity range-of-motion exercises every hour while awake. To make this a more interesting task for the patient, a small beach ball can be placed at the foot of the bed and the patient instructed to press it with his toes and move it with his feet. It also helps to keep pressure from the bed linens off the toes and reminds the patient to keep his legs uncrossed.

When the patient is ready to sit on the side of the bed or get out of bed to a chair, blood pressure response should be carefully monitored. Blood pressure readings should be taken prior to the activity and immediately after. The development of orthostatic hypotension is always a possibility. Support

Level	1	2	3
Feed self			
Wash face and hands, brush teeth			
Deep breathing	Every hour while awake		
Bed commode (3 METS)			
Dangle	Passive, 3 times a day	Active, every hour while awake	
Leg and ankle activity			
Partial bath, self-grooming			
Chair at bedside		Once a day	Twice a day
Meals in chair			Breakfast
Ambulate in area of bed			

☐ Appropriate ▓ Not Appropriate

Figure 3-3. Recommended Phase I activities (1 to 2 METs). (For a discussion of METs, see Chapter 6.)

37

stockings should be left on. The feet should be supported if the patient is to dangle or should be able to rest flat on the floor if he is to sit in a chair. The patient's back should be supported and a place provided to rest his arms.

When the patient first stands at the bedside, he should not be permitted to remain stationary. He should be instructed to move his leg muscles in some manner, such as walking slowly in place. This movement will facilitate venous return from the legs and help prevent development of hypotension. The blood pressure should be carefully monitored the first time the patient stands at the bedside, and the patient should be carefully observed for any signs of intolerance.

Early Education and Psychological Support

Orientation to and reassurance about CCU surroundings and events should be part of planned nursing care for every acute cardiac patient. As the patient is being admitted, careful explanation of admission procedures, such as IVs, ECGs, oxygen, and monitoring equipment should be offered in an effort to lower anxiety. Demonstration of the cardiac alarm system and explanation that alarms are frequently triggered by movement, loose "patches," and so on should be offered so that the patient is not overwhelmed by thinking that every bell he hears is an emergency.

To prevent misinterpretation that his condition is worse, routines of checking vital signs and monitor readings should be explained. A display of competence on the part of the staff will help the patient feel more secure and less anxious. In addition, the patient should be assured that his significant others will be informed about his condition and treatment and that they will be given whatever help they need to handle this unexpected event.

Emphasis should be on the positive: the constant availability of the nursing staff, the "early warning systems" of the various monitoring devices, and the expectation of recovery.

Patients may be helped by knowing that feelings of anxiety in this situation are quite normal. The nurse should be watchful for signs of anxiety, confirm her observation with the patient, and then offer specific reassurances. For example, if the patient appears apprehensive about getting out of bed for the first time, he should be questioned. If it is confirmed that the patient is fearful, the nurse can offer specific reassurances. Many times patients have a misconception about their disease and treatment which can be the source of anxiety. In the above example, the patient may remember that treatment for myocardial infarction not many years ago was strict bed rest for a period of weeks. He may not realize that this is no longer the treatment of choice or understand the benefits of early ambulation.

The unknown can be much more terrifying than the understood. Misconceptions and erroneous knowledge can keep a patient in a state of anxiety. Patients should be asked what they understand about their situation. Information should either be confirmed or corrected in an effort to help patients adjust.

Daily positive feedback on progress, offered to both the patient and family will help them maintain a realistic view of the problem. Probably the most effective method of demonstrating to the patient and family that he is in the process of recovery is the addition of activities to his daily routine and evidence that these increased functions are tolerated without difficulty.

Patients and family should be prepared for the feeling of weakness nearly every cardiac patient experiences. Weakness is especially distressing for the patient who had an image of himself as a strong person prior to the acute event. An explanation that this is normal, that early activity will help maintain present strength, and that cardiac patients can return to a state of vigor equal to or greater than that enjoyed previously may help avert feelings of depression likely to accompany weakness.

The patient in CCU may be plagued by the question of having the ability to have sex again. Male patients often perceive a heart attack as a threat to masculinity. At this time, the patient may not be ready for an in-depth discussion concerning return to sexual activity, but the nurse should attempt to allay his fears and furnish information he may request.

Providing models of people who have led and who continue to lead active and productive lives after experiencing heart attacks is encouraging to some patients. Actor Walter Matthau and Presidents Johnson and Eisenhower are familiar examples.

Most reports indicate that both anxiety and depression are reduced in patients actively engaged in rehabilitation programs. Patients able to participate in their recovery experience a restored confidence when it is demonstrated that activity is possible.[9]

(Patient ID Stamp) C. P.			CARDIAC REHAB CARE PLAN	
Date Identified	**Need/Problem**	**Approach**	**Behavioral Objectives**	**Date Achieved Changed**
5/1/XX	**Physiological**		The patient will be able to	
	1. prevent decon- ditioning 2. begin self-care	1. ⎫ begin Phase 1 ⎬ activity levels 2. ⎭ with MD orders	1. ⎫ gradually increase self- ⎬ care and physical 2. ⎭ activities (per Phase I sequence) without undue responses.	
	Psychosocial			
	3. fear of dying (implied)	3. facilitate discussion of feelings; pro- vide frequent reassurance of CCU purpose; offer availability of mental health nurse specialist and clergyman	3. within the next 24-48 hours express his fear of dying and openly commun- icate related anxieties (concerns re family, farm, finances, etc.)	
	4. anxiety re farm work	4. discuss options with patient and family re tempo- rary help— family, friends; contact social service	4. arrange for outside help within the next 2-3 days	

(Patient ID Stamp)

C. P.

**CARDIAC REHAB
CARE PLAN**

Date Identified	Need/Problem	Approach	Behavioral Objectives	Date Achieved Changed
(adm. cont.)	**Educational**		The patient will be able to	
	5. lacks awareness of heart attack and healing (seems to think	5. patient and family educa- tion session "What is a Heart	5. prior to transfer from CCU a) describe what a heart attack is in his own words	
	death is inevit- able, recovery rare)	Attack" with heart model and textbook pictures	b) indicate the area of his occlusion on a heart diagram	
			c) illustrate healing on the diagram	
	6. needs to know rehab is planned (because recov- ery is expected)	6. description of rehab program, emphasizing	6. in 2-3 days a) describe purpose of gradual increases in activity	
	and how it will proceed	activity increases	b) express interest in rehab program participation through questions re	
			progress	

(Patient ID Stamp) C. P.	PHYSICIANS' ORDER SHEET
Date/Time	**ORDERS**
5/1/XX 10 a.m.	(routine admission orders)
(on admission)	Have cardiac rehab nurse consult
	J. D., M.D.
5/2/XX 8 a.m.	
(day following admission)	Begin Phase I cardiac rehab program, with progressive activity levels, heart rate limit at 100.
	J. D. M.D.

References

1. WALTER, J. D., PARDEE, G. P., and MOLBO, D. M., *Dynamics of Problem-Oriented Approaches: Patient Care and Documentation* (Philadelphia: J. B. Lippincott Company, 1976), p. 20.
2. WENGER, N. K., *Coronary Care: Rehabilitation After Myocardial Infarction* (New York: American Heart Association, 1973), p. 6.
3. *Ibid*, pp. 18-25.
4. JOHNSTON, B. L., CANTWELL, J. D., and FLETCHER, G. F., "Eight Steps to Inpatient Cardiac Rehabilitation: The Team Effort—Methodology and Preliminary Results," *Heart and Lung*, January-February 1976, pp. 97-111.
5. BARRY, E. M., KNIGHT, S. A., and ACKER, J. E., "Hospital Program for Cardiac Rehabilitation," *American Journal of Nursing*, December 1972, pp. 2174-2177.
6. THE NORTH CAROLINA HEART ASSOCIATION, *Organizational Guidelines for Myocardial Infarction Rehabilitation Program* (Chapel Hill, North Carolina: The North Carolina Heart Association, 1974), pp. 25-26.
7. LAWSON, M., "Progressive Coronary Care," *Heart and Lung*, March-April 1972, pp. 240-253.
8. CIUCA, R., BRADISH, J., and TROMBLY, S. M., "Passive Range-of-Motion Exercises," *Nursing 78*, July, pp. 59-65.
9. WENGER, *op. cit.*, p. 8.

4

implementation of phase I cardiac rehabilitation

Behavioral Objectives

After completion of this chapter, the reader should be able to:

- define "implementation" and discuss its significance in the nursing process.

- discuss general influences to be considered in implementing cardiac rehab care.

- propose a method of charting for cardiac rehab practice and list the types of records needed to document rehab care.

- identify which nurses have responsibility for Phase I rehabilitation in the reader's own practice setting.

Introduction

Implementation is the conversion of a finished plan into action. It is planning made visible, the actual doing of what has been thought out by the nurse and talked over with the patient. Implementation can be defined as the initiation and completion of actions necessary to accomplish objectives.[1]

Responsibility for executing the plan, built upon earlier assessments, belongs to the nurse. Actions taken may include performing technical procedures, coordinating the services of or collaborating with other health professionals, directing or supervising the patient's self-care, and conducting educational programs. To be effective, implemented nursing actions must be performed competently and conscientiously.

General Considerations for Implementing Cardiac Rehabilitation

The purpose of the fourth chapter in each unit is to identify influences on implementation of individualized rehab care plans as well as influences affecting conduction of the cardiac rehabilitation program as a whole.

The Cardiac Rehab Service

Taking action as instructed on a well-written rehab care plan seems a direct and an easy task. However, since nursing practice in cardiac rehabilitation usually exists as part of a larger health care operation, one additional planning step precedes action. Consideration must be given to how the guidelines and regulations of the total organization affect plans for cardiac rehabilitation.

As mentioned in Chapter 1, organizational policies influence nursing functions. Since implementation is the most tangible step in the nursing process organizational influences are frequently manifested as action begins. Basic influences that guide and shape cardiac rehabilitation programs are illustrated in Figure 4-1. Such influences are automatically considered during planning once programs are firmly established.

The four phases of the rehab process occur in two divisions of health care: inpatient hospital care, and outpatient care associated with either a hospital medical clinic or an ambulatory care agency. Usually, one set of organizational guidelines presides over the inpatient program and another over the outpatient program. Both programs may have many points of operation in common, especially if located in the same institution and managed by the same team, or they may be independent and distinct. Chapters 9 and 19 detail inpatient and outpatient organizational concerns respectively, while Chapters 4, 9, 14, and 19 present specific operational considerations for each phase.

The Cardiac Rehab Record

A major part of "doing" in nursing practice is documenting what has been done and what effect it has had. Nursing, like other health professions, has been inundated with paper, the meaning and usefulness of which is often questioned. Formats for nursing records are abundant.

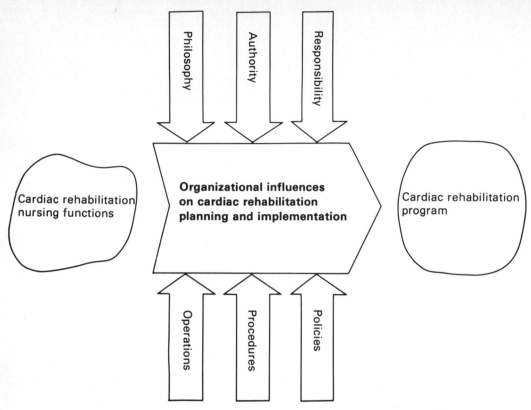

Figure 4-1. Organizational influences in cardiac rehabilitation.

Charting Method. One approach which improves use of health care records and provides a universal recording format is the system of problem-oriented medical records (POMR). The POMR method of charting was popularized in the 1960s by Lawrence Weed.[2]

Complete description of the POMR system is not within the scope of this text; however, the format utilized by the system for charting is the method of choice for cardiac rehab record entries. Identified by the acronym SOAP, the format divides notations into four related components: Subjective data, Objective data, Assessment, and Plan.

In the original system, each letter of SOAP is separately correlated to each of the patient's problems by an identifying number. All health professionals caring for the patient record their findings on the same patient record using the SOAP format. The charting examples presented in this text are shown in a modified problem-oriented format which can easily be expanded to fit the formal POMR or integrated into traditional nursing notes to enhance charting consistency and encourage entries more descriptive and meaningful than those written in the past. Table 4-1 provides samples of nurses' notes that have been recorded using SOAP. Additional examples are included in the sample case at the end of the chapters.

Table 4-1
SOAP in Cardiac Rehab Charting

Outline	Inpatient Example	Outpatient Example
Charting format:	Date, 8:30 A.M.	Date, 2 P.M.
S = Subjective information: what the patient says, what his comments or actions imply, the attitude he displays, and so on.	During A.M. nursing rounds on step down unit patients, this patient in the unit since yesterday, complained of chest discomfort for the first time since transfer.	Patient arrived for usual exercise session.
	S = "I got a tight ache in my chest just after breakfast" (20 minutes ago).	S = Volunteered the information that he started smoking again. "Everyone on the job takes cigarette breaks. I was the only one not smoking." Seems upset about giving in to this weakness.
O = Objective information: nursing observations, physical appraisal findings, measurements taken, results of studies, and so on.	O = Pale, slightly diaphoretic, rubbing midsternal area. Telemetry monitor shows 6-10 VPCs/min. HR at 90. S³ on auscultation. B/P 104/60. STAT 12 lead ECG shows elevated ST segments V_2 - V_5.	O = Pre-exercise HR at 88, usually 70-75. No other unusual pre-exercise findings. Lungs clear. Heart rate responses to exercise exaggerated. Decreased work so as not to exceed training heart rate.
A = Assessment: conclusion drawn from subjective and objective input.	A = May be extending anterior MI.	A = Higher-than-usual HR responses probably due to recent resumption of cigarette smoking.
P = Plan: action(s) to be taken.	P = Notify physician, start lidocaine drip, transfer back to CCU, explain to patient and family, and offer support through new crisis.	P = Show patient response changes and discuss cause. Suggest he reconsider his smoking. Recommend community withdrawal program for added support.
	D. N., R.N.	*N. T.*, R.N.

Rehab Records. To minimize paper requirements while optimizing charting usefulness, the following types of forms are recommended for standard use in cardiac rehabilitation nursing. Most are applicable in either inpatient or outpatient rehab settings.

Assessment Records. Multiple assessments are inherent in cardiac rehab nursing practice. Some require in-depth interview of the patient while others include specific examinations. Outlines that serve as reminders of points to be covered, information to be collected, measurements to be taken, and so on are useful during assessment procedures. Results can be documented on records keyed to major assessment categories. Outpatient nursing history, nutritional history, cardiovascular examination, and chest pain assessment are among the assessment guidelines discussed here.

Care Plans. As discussed in Chapter 3, some form of documentation is necessary to outline assessment results as needs and problems, to express nursing actions to be taken, and to define patient results to be expected. The rehab care plan is basic to all cardiac rehab nursing. Samples are shown at the end of each planning chapter.

Progress Notes. Becknell and Smith define a progress note as a written record describing developments in a predetermined plan of nursing care.[3] In cardiac rehab practice, the nurses' progress notes provide information about the patient's admission, his responses to specific therapy, new problems that develop, needs that are met, and transfer or discharge. Progress note entries utilize the SOAP method. The case report provides examples.

Flow Sheets. Rehab-related events requiring extensive or frequent data collection are best reported on specific flow sheets. Flow sheets are correlated with progress notes. Entries should be complementary: the flow sheet presenting the data, the progress note providing amplification or explanation of the flow sheet. Flow sheet samples for exercise stress testing, inpatient activity progression, and outpatient exercise training are included in this book.

Implementing a Phase I Program

Rehabilitative action in CCU sets the pace for all cardiac rehab efforts to follow. Structurally, Phase I is the entry level of a comprehensive inpatient cardiac rehabilitation program. As such, Phase I efforts are usually directed by the same guidelines defining Phase II operations (See Chapter 9).

Questions most specific to implementation of a Phase I program include the following:

- Which professionals have primary responsibility for rehab care in the acute unit? The critical care nurse responsible for direct patient care? The cardiac rehab nurse specialist responsible for inpatient rehab? The primary care nurse with total patient responsibility?
- Are staffing patterns conducive to rehab functions which often require "quiet time" for just being with the patient and/or family?
- What medical direction is required for rehab functions? Does each rehab effort need a specific order or can selected functions be included with CCU standing orders for "when stable," for examples bedside commode, beach ball, and so on?

Given the answers to these questions and the knowledge of what should be done, why, and how, as discussed in preceding chapters, Phase I cardiac rehab should be a recognizable part of CCU care.

(Patient ID Stamp)	
C. P.	**CARDIAC REHAB PROGRESS NOTES**

Date/Time	PROGRESS NOTES
5/2/XX 9 a.m.	Phase I/Level 1:
	S. "I feel O.K. . . . will be glad to do something!" Still not too talkative.
	O. No abnormal heart or lung sounds. Afebrile, other vital signs on activity.
	flow sheet. A.M. ECG shows bi-phasic T waves II, III, AVF. No rhythm
	abnormalities since admission.
	A. No inappropriate responses to passive ROM. Explained ROM exercises and
	rationale. Deep breathing encouraged.
	P. Will repeat passive ROM this P.M. and have patient describe purpose of
	regular leg exercises. Active ROM and beach ball exercises for tomorrow.
	N. S. R.N.

CARDIAC ACTIVITY PROGRESSION FLOW SHEET

Name ____   Phase I   **Physician** ____

C. P.   J. D.

	HR	Preactivity Rhythm	Preactivity BP	Activity Performed	HR	Activity Response Rhythm	Activity Response BP	HR	Postactivity Rhythm	Postactivity BP	Supervised By
Date: 5/2/XX **Level:** 1				**Rx Date:** 5/2/XX **HR Limit:** 100							
Time 9 a.m.	80	NSR	140/80	Passive leg and ankle exercises	84	NSR	142/76	80	NSR	138/80	n.J., R.N.
Time 2:30 p.m.	76	NSR	132/74	Passive leg and ankle exercises	80	NSR	132/70	78	NSR	132/70	n.J., R.N.
Time 7:30 p.m.	84	NSR	130/70	Passive leg and ankle exercises	84	NSR	134/70	82	NSR	134/70	n.J., R.N.
Date: 5/3/XX **Level:** 2				**Rx Date:** 5/3/XX **HR Limit:** 100							
Time 10 a.m.	82	NSR	132/82	Bedside chair	86	NSR	136/84	84	NSR	130/80	n.J., R.N.
Time 2 p.m.	80	NSR	130/76	Active leg and ankle movements	84	NSR	134/76	82	NSR	130/84	n.J., R.N.
Time											
Date: **Level:**				**HR Limit:**							
Time											
Time											
Time											
Date: **Level:**				**HR Limit:**							
Time											
Time											
Time											
Date: **Level:**				**HR Limit:**							
Time											
Time											
Time											
Date: **Level:**				**HR Limit:**							
Time											
Time											
Time											

References

1. GANONG, J. M. and GANONG, W. L., *Nursing Management* (Germantown, Maryland: Aspen Systems Corporation, 1976), p. 53.
2. WEED, L. L., *Medical Records, Medical Education, and Patient Care* (Chicago, Illinois: The Press of Case Western Reserve University, Cleveland/Year Book Medical Publishers, Inc. 1969).
3. BECKNELL, E. P. and SMITH, D. M., *System of Nursing Practice* (Philadelphia: F. A. Davis Company, 1975), p. 103.

5

evaluation of phase I cardiac rehabilitation

Behavioral Objectives

After completion of this chapter, the reader should be able to:
- define "evaluation" and discuss its significance in the nursing process.
- describe the types of evaluation useful in determining the effectiveness of cardiac rehab nursing.
- define "patient outcome" and discuss the usefulness of an outcome approach to evaluation.
- list at least four patient outcomes to be expected from an effective Phase I program.
- name at least three sources of transfer-related anxiety.

Introduction

Evaluation can be thought of as the process of gathering information to ascertain the value of something.[1] As the fourth step in the nursing process, evaluation involves the review of cardiac rehab nursing care rendered and the determination of its effect on the patient. Self-evaluation and peer review of nursing effectiveness are basic to professional accountability.

Evaluating Cardiac Rehabilitation Nursing Care: An Overview

In cardiac rehabilitation nursing practice, evaluation must address both specific patient results and general program performance. The purpose of the fifth chapter in each unit is to offer suggestions as to how effectiveness may be determined. The following overview is provided to emphasize evaluation applications.

Types of Evaluation

Although generally interpreted as an end-stage occurrence, a look at things past, evaluation of cardiac rehab nursing care should occur in three different time frames.

Short-Term Evaluation. It is a nursing responsibility to assess the patient's progress with each rehab encounter. Responses should show evidence that the rehab plan is working. In other words, planning effectiveness is being evaluated each time the nurse sees the patient. If responses are not as desired, the plan is judged ineffective and adjustments made to improve results. This ongoing type of evaluation is called concurrent review—the evaluation occurs at the same time the plan is being implemented.

Intermediate Evaluation. Each phase of cardiac rehabilitation is a link in a comprehensive sequential process, or continuum. The results of care in one phase influence the plans for care in the next. Evaluation of the effectiveness of rehab care given in each phase is performed as the patient approaches phase completion. This retrospective, or postimplementation, review determines if the patient achieved the health status for which rehab care during the phase was intended. Effectiveness at this intermediate rehab level is best judged by examining the patient's behavioral changes, or "outcomes," resulting from cardiac rehabilitation nursing care during that phase (see Patient Outcomes, page 54).

Long-Term Evaluation. The cumulative results of the successive rehab phases determine the outcome of the rehab process as a whole. Achievement of optimal health can be evaluated based on additive outcomes upon completion of the cardiac rehab continuum. However, maintenance of optimal health, the coequal ultimate rehab goal, can only be determined over an extended period. Follow-up should be arranged to allow opportunity for this long-term evaluation.

Program Results

As a functioning health care entity, the cardiac rehab program itself needs to be evaluated for effectiveness and efficiency. Program effectiveness is directly related to patient results. That is, if the majority of patients achieve the goals for which the program was intended, the program is considered effective.

Program efficiency is usually determined through review from two other points of view. Structure evaluation looks at the things a program must have to work well. For example, "every cardiac rehab area must have complete cardiac emergency equipment on site." The structure evaluation is the approach used by most inspection committees and agencies.

Process evaluation examines what the cardiac rehab nurse must do, or the activities she must perform, for the program to work well. For example, "cardiac rehab nurses will use telemetry to monitor all exercises performed by cardiac patients." The process evaluation is the approach used for many nursing audits.

A successful program is a combination of effectiveness and efficiency, both highly dependent upon professional nursing performance.

Patient Outcomes

Planning of cardiac rehab care incorporates the purpose and goals of each rehab phase into patient objectives. As discussed in Chapter 3, an objective is a projection of a desired end, a statement of a goal. An outcome is the result of an action. It is the alteration in the health status of the patient caused by goal-directed patient care activities.[2] Ideally, the objectives become the outcomes with the result that the two words are frequently used synonymously. In this text, the term "objective" is used in a prospective sense and "outcome" in a retrospective sense to distinguish "before and after" applications.

Individual results of rehab care, or outcomes, can be readily determined at the end of each rehab phase by reviewing objectives. Did the patient accomplish the behavior that was specified in the objectives? Was the behavior performed to a satisfactory degree? If not, why? What could have been done differently? What can be done now?

Once a specific patient's outcomes are determined, it is of further value to compare his achievements to those of other myocardial infarction patients with similar problems completing the phase of care being evaluated. Just as common nursing goals can be formulated based on patient similarities (See Chapter 3), common patient outcomes can be constructed for use as a general reference to compare the results of rehab care. Common patient outcomes presented in the evaluation chapters of this text can provide the basic rehab criteria for formal audits based on patient outcomes.

Evaluation of Patient Responses to Phase I

Determination of Outcomes

Although Phase I has the shortest duration of the four phases in the cardiac rehab sequence, it's first place position makes effective rehab care during this three- to five-day period imperative. Effectiveness is best evaluated by determining the outcomes of rehab care rendered in CCU.

As the patient is awaiting transfer, determination should be made of which of the objectives specified in the patient's rehab care plan have been achieved during Phase I and which remain to be transferred to Phase II. Such identification of behavioral change requires subjective input from the patient and objective analysis by the nurse. If objectives were realistically planned and if the plan was adjusted as responses warranted, most Phase I patients will have achieved the common patient outcomes shown in Table 5-1 prior to transfer.

Table 5-1
Common Patient Outcomes of Phase I Cardiac Rehabilitation

Physiological Outcomes

Upon completion of the Phase I inpatient program, the cardiac patient should be able to:
Display none of the complications of bed rest.
Perform basic self-care activities without negative effects.

Psychosocial Outcomes

Upon completion of the Phase I inpatient program, the cardiac patient should be able to:
Accept his diagnosis of myocardial infarction as evidenced by a statement that he has had a heart attack, discussion of necessary life adjustments with significant others.
Begin to express his feelings about this unexpected change in health status.

Educational Outcomes

Upon completion of the Phase I inpatient program, the cardiac patient should be able to:
Correctly describe a heart attack and discuss the healing process in his own words.
Give the basic reasons for gradual, guided activity resumption.
Freely ask questions about what he's experiencing and the care he is receiving.

Preparation for Transfer

Transfer is a rehab event as well as a patient experience. Since transfer marks stepping from one rehab phase to another, preparation for transfer should be viewed as a rehab responsibility.

Transfer from CCU is a major anxiety-producing change for post-myocardial infarction patients.[3] Nursing efforts to minimize perceived threats accompanying transfer should include education emphasizing the following positive points:

- Transfer is a benchmark in the recovery process since the medical decision to move the patient from the CCU reflects ability to progress.
- Even though there are fewer eyes and fewer machines constantly observing the patient, capable staff members are always nearby and can be summoned in an instant.
- The same cardiac rehab nurse specialist already known to the patient in Phase I will continue to work with him in his new location.

Transfer should be as carefully planned as any rehab activity. If at all possible, "emergency transfers" should be avoided since they are usually

	(Patient ID Stamp)	
	C. P.	**CARDIAC REHAB PROGRESS NOTES**

Date/Time	PROGRESS NOTES
5/5/XX 11 a.m.	To be transferred to PCCU after lunch. Phase I Rehab summary: Objectives 1, 2, 4, 5, 6 achieved as noted on Rehab Plan. Objective 3 to be continued into Phase II.
	S. Patient was fearful and extremely anxious at times during CCU stay. Lessened as transfer approached. Stated he'll "return to my teaching job and farm work by fall." Although fear resurfaces occasionally, "if I make it home."
	O. With initial activity progression B/P was 140/80 due to anxiety. No abnormal responses during Phase I activities. Rhythm remained NSR, no ectopics. ECG shows biphasic T waves II, III, AVF.
	A. Patient did well in Phase I rehab, has a good knowledge base and is motivated to continue Phase II.
	P. Will assist with transfer and introductions to PCCU staff.
	N. S., R.N.

accompanied by several unknowns—Where can we get a bed for this patient? What's the new patient's condition?—creating anxiety in both patient and staff members.

Advising the patient and significant others of the expected transfer time and detaching monitors in advance provides reassurance of cardiac stability and allows time for questions to be answered and change accepted. A partial solution to the problem of transfer anxiety is the availability of an intermediate unit to receive patients transferred from CCU.[4]

References

1. PHANEUF, M. C., *The Nursing Audit,* 2nd ed. (New York: Appleton-Century-Crofts, 1976), p. 149.
2. ZIMMER, M. J., "Quality Assurance for Nursing Care," *Quality Assurance for Nursing Care* (Proceedings of an Institute), American Nurses' Association, 1976), p. 4.
3. HACKETT, T. P., and CASSEM, N. H., *Coronary Care: Patient Psychology* (New York: American Heart Association, 1975), p. 9.
4. *Ibid.*

unit II

phase II cardiac rehabilitation

6

background and basics of phase II cardiac rehabilitation

Behavioral Objectives

After completion of this chapter, the reader should be able to:
- **state the purpose and benefits of a Phase II cardiac rahab program.**
- **identify specialized nursing knowledge needed for Phase II practice.**
- **relate the sequence of normal oxygen transport.**
- **define MET and explain use of MET values in cardiac rehab.**
- **define isometric and isotonic exercise, give at least six examples of each, and summarize the respective underlying physiology.**

Introduction

Upon leaving the CCU, the patient may find himself in an "intermediate cardiac care unit," a "progressive unit," or a "step down unit," each title an alias for the same place—a special nursing unit designed to receive patients from the acute CCU. Although, length of stay in the acute and postacute units is a matter for individualized physician judgment, patients with uncomplicated myocardial infarction usually spend three to five days in the acute unit, then are transferred to the progressive unit for the next ten to fourteen days. Transfer marks the beginning of a Phase II cardiac rehabilitation program.

Purpose

A Phase II cardiac rehab program is a head start toward the cardiac rehab goal of optimal health. Phase II continues the purpose of rehab initiated in Phase I: to minimize the negative physical and psychological effects of acute myocardial infarction. In Phase II, efforts to prevent deconditioning and provide psychological support are intensified through graduated activity progression and an organized educational program. Emphasis on self-care and activities of daily living contributes to regaining independence so that the patient will not feel helpless upon discharge.

It has been well documented that activity performed within the physiological capabilities of the patient can, to a great extent, prevent the effects of deconditioning, while at the same time not increasing morbidity as measured by ventricular dysrhythmias, aneurysm, congestive heart failure, or recurrence of chest pain.[1-8] Another significant benefit for myocardial infarction patients who have the advantage of participating in inpatient rehabilitation programs as stated by the American Heart Association is ". . . an improved quality of life for the survivors of AMI and an increased ability to more rapidly return to work."[9]

Nursing Requisites

As discussed in Chapter 1, cardiac rehab nursing requires an advanced level of knowledge and capability to use related skills. Basic requirements for effective Phase II nursing are shown in Table 6-1. Phase II nursing functions are detailed in succeeding chapters.

Physiological Basis

Prevention of deconditioning, the adverse physical state precipitated by inactivity, can be accomplished safely by a well-supervised, gradually increased activity program. Basic to the structure of an appropriate program is an understanding of the following physiological principles.

Normal Oxygen Transport

The key to optimal physical health is the body's ability to take in, transport, and use a sufficient amount of oxygen to carry out whatever task is at hand. Normal oxygen transport occurs in a sequence of events that can be conveniently, albeit simplistically, listed in alphabetical order for easy recall and correlation (See Table 6-2).

Table 6-1
Specialized Nursing Requirements for Phase II Cardiac Rehabilitation

Cognitive	Psychomotor

Principles of teaching/learning
Educational techniques
  Methods
  Aids
Physiological basis of progressive
activity
  Methods of exercise progression
  Potential benefits and hazards
Principles of predischarge
exercise testing
	Performance of activity levels
	Use of telemetry
	Audiovisual equipment operation
	for patient education

Table 6-2
Systemic Oxygen Transport

A: Air	Oxygen makes up nearly 21 percent of the earth's atmosphere. As long as air is available, oxygen is supplied in sufficient amounts.
B: Breathing	Oxygen is taken into the lungs through the mechanical action of respiration. Upon reaching the alveolar level, oxygen diffuses into the bloodstream. The amount of oxygen received by the blood depends upon the integrity of the pulmonary system.
C: Circulation	Oxygen carried in the blood is delivered to all parts of the body through cardiac pumping action. Should this action be disrupted, delivery will be impaired and some degree of damage may result.
D: Diffusion	Oxygen carried by hemoglobin and in blood plasma arrives at the cellular level and diffuses into each cell in needed amounts. Insufficient amounts of hemoglobin, as in anemia, result in decreased availability of oxygen for diffusion.
E: Energy	Oxygen provides the source of cellular energy. Mitochondria require oxygen for aerobic metabolism to produce energy. When insufficient oxygen is available metabolism proceeds under anerobic conditions creating acid by-products.
F: Follow-through	Oxygen not used, along with carbon dioxide, is returned to the lungs through the venous system.

The amount of oxygen the body needs to carry out its functions at minimal levels has been measured as 3.5 ml. of oxygen per Kg. of body weight per minute.[10] This value is essentially a resting metabolic rate. To explain, for a 100 Kg. (220 lb.) man to sit relaxed in a chair for one minute, he needs to take in and transport 3.5 ml. of oxygen per Kg. or a total of 350 ml. of oxygen. Under the same conditions, a 50 Kg. (110 lb.) woman would also need 3.5 ml. per Kg. per minute, but her total oxygen used would be 175 ml.

Logically, it follows that any increase in activity from the relative resting state just described requires an increase in oxygen transport. Instead of the cumbersome value X ml. per Kg. per minute to express amounts of oxygen, the extent of increase can be expressed more usefully as multiples of the 3.5 ml. per Kg. per minute resting level. Assigning a value of 1 to the resting level would mean that twice that level would be equivalent to 7.0 ml. per Kg. per minute, three times would equal 10.5 ml. per Kg. per minute, five times 17.5 ml. per Kg. per minute, eight times 28.0 ml. per Kg. per minute, and so on. These multiples of resting oxygen levels are called metabolic equivalents, or METs.[11]

Physiologists and medical scientists have investigated and measured oxygen transport in a number of therapeutic, occupational, and recreational activities. A number of tables are available for organizing the results of such studies into MET categories.[12-14] The MET equivalents are a practical objective guideline for physical performance in various rehab settings.

As discussed in Chapter 3, activities recommended for CCU are in the one-to-two-MET range. In Phase II, activities gradually increase until most patients are able to perform at a three-to-four-MET level by discharge. In general, performance levels achieved in Phase II correspond to the energy level of most daily activities, including many household and job tasks.

Types of Exercise

Activities for the postmyocardial infarction patient must be carefully selected so as not to further jeopardize an already impaired oxygen transport system. Low-level activity is one safety consideration. A second choice influencing oxygen transport is the type of exercise. For the purposes of cardiac rehab, two types of exercise must be understood.

Isometric Exercise. Isometric exercise is an activity that involves muscle contraction without movement. More technically, contraction is isometric when both ends of a muscle are fixed so that no significant shortening can occur.[15] The classic isometric example is the weight lifting press—suspending hundreds of pounds of iron above one's head is the epitome of still life muscle contraction.

On a daily basis, isometric activities can usually be identified as those that involve pushing, pulling, lifting, or carrying. Familiar examples include carrying bags of groceries or baskets of wash, hanging heavy wash items (blankets, towels) on a line, shoveling snow, carrying luggage, or moving furniture. Activities performed with the arms overhead are, in effect, isometric, since arm weight, in addition to any weight involved with the task, is lifted and supported. Washing windows, painting walls, and ceilings, and placing items on high shelves are examples. Some sport and recreational activities that are heavily isometric because of sustained muscle contraction are water skiing, horseback riding, and sailing.

The physiological changes resulting from isometric activity are reason for concern with cardiac patients. Isometric contraction inhibits blood flow and, thus, oxygen transport to muscles. Peripheral resistance is increased and, in turn, left ventricular pressure and systolic blood pressure are elevated. This sudden "pressure overload" on the left ventricle increases myocardial oxygen need in an already compromised coronary delivery system and the potential end result is an ischemic complication, such as lethal arrhythmia or extended infarction.

Isometrics, also called "static" exercises, are, therefore, inappropriate for rehab activities. In early stages of recovery, special nursing efforts are needed to help patients avoid self-induced isometric activities like pushing themselves up in bed or performing a Valsalva maneuver (practically unavoidable if bedpans are used for bowel movements).

Isotonic Exercise. In contrast, isotonic exercise is activity that requires alternate degrees of muscle contraction. The muscle fibers vary their length during contraction.[16] Characterized by motion, walking-jogging-running activities are the traditional examples.

Everyday activities that involve repeated, fairly smooth motion, such as walking the dog or running to catch the commuter train are isotonic. In addition to a host of popular walking-running activities, swimming, cycling, and dancing are excellent recreational isotonics. Basketball and tennis are sports that are mainly isotonic.

Performance of isotonic activities may enhance cardiovascular efficiency through "volume overload" of the left ventricle. As muscles perform rhythmic movement, additional oxygen is required by the working muscle cells. Through an increase in heart rate and stroke volume, cardiac output is increased. Vasodilatation occurs in the working muscles and a greater oxygen supply is delivered. (See Chapter 16 for a detailed description of oxygen transport adaptations to exercise.)

An increase in venous return results from the pumping action of working muscles on the veins coupled with the thoracic suction effect of increased respiration. Greater volume passes through the right heart, pulmonary circulation, and into the left heart. When this increased amount of blood reaches the left ventricle, it causes muscle fibers to stretch in order to contain the greater volume in the chamber. This left ventricular distention activates the Frank-Starling mechanism, whereby muscle fibers stretched farther contract harder, producing greater emptying of the ventricle. Over time, this effect may result in an improved stroke volume.[17]

Isotonics are the exercises of choice for cardiac patients. "Dynamic" activities are used throughout the cardiac rehab process, beginning with walking in the room while still in CCU, to walking stairs before discharge, to treadmill exercise testing, to daily jogging, and on a rare occasion to a very special cardiac rehab patient who completes the Boston marathon![18]

Table 6-3 compares isometric and isotonic effects.

Table 6-3
Comparison of Isometric and Isotonic Effects

The *Hazard* of Isometric Activity	The *Benefit* of Isotonic Activity
Isometric contraction	Isotonic movement
↓	↓
Restricts arterial flow	Increases cardiac output
↓	↓
Increases peripheral resistance	Increases vasodilatation
↓	↓
Increases left ventricular pressure	Increases venous return
↓	↓
Increases systolic blood pressure	Increases left ventricular distention
↓	↓
Increases myocardial oxygen demand	Increases force of contraction
↓	↓
May cause serious cardiac complications	May result in improved stroke volume

References

1. GRODEN, B. M., ALLISON, A., and SHAW, G. B., "Management of Myocardial Infarction, The Effect of Early Mobilization," *Scottish Medical Journal*, Vol. 12, 1967, pp. 435-440.
2. HARPUR, J. E., et al., "Controlled Trial of Early Mobilization and Discharge From Hospital in Uncomplicated Myocardial Infarction," *Lancet*, Vol. 2, 1971, pp. 1331-1334.
3. HUTTER, A. M., and SIDEL, V. W., et al., "Early Discharge After Myocardial Infarction," *New England Journal of Medicine*, Vol. 228, 1973, pp. 1141-1144.
4. LAMERS, H. J. and DROST, W. S., et al., "Early Mobilization After Myocardial Infarction: A Controlled Study" *British Medical Journal*, Vol. 1, 1973, pp. 257-259.
5. GLASGOW ROYAL INFIRMARY, "Early Mobilization After Uncomplicated Myocardial Infarction," *Lancet*, Vol. 2, 1973, pp. 346-349.
6. HAYES, M. J., MORRIS, G. K. and JAMPTON, J. R., "Comparison of Mobilization After Two and Nine Days in Uncomplicated Myocardial Infarction," *British Medical Journal*, Vol. 3, 1973, pp. 10-13.
7. BLOCH, A. and MARDER, J. P., et al., "Early Mobilization After Myocardial Infarction: A Controlled Study," *American Journal of Cardiology*, Vol. 34, 1974, pp. 152-157.
8. ABRAHAM, A. S. and SEVER, Y., et al., "Value of Early Ambulation in Patients With and Without Complications After Acute Myocardial Infarction," *New England Journal of Medicine*, Vol. 292, 1975, pp. 719-722.
9. WENGER, N. K., *Coronary Care—Rehabilitation After Myocardial Infarction* (New York: American Heart Association, 1973), p. 15.
10. CARDIAC RECONDITIONING and WORK EVALUATION UNIT, *Exercise Equivalents* (Denver, Colorado: Colorado Heart Association, 1970), pp. 1-3.
11. *Ibid.*
12. AMERICAN COLLEGE of SPORTS MEDICINE, *Guidelines for Graded Exercise Testing and Exercise Prescription* (Philadelphia: Lea & Febiger, 1975), Tables 9-11.
13. COMMITTEE on EXERCISE, *Exercise Testing and Training of Individuals with Heart Disease or at High Risk for its Development: A Handbook for Physicians* (New York: American Heart Association, 1975), Table 4.
14. CARDIAC RECONDITIONING and WORK EVALUATION UNIT, *op. cit.*, pp. 1-24.
15. NUTTER, D. O., SCHLANT, R. C., and HURST, J. W., "Isometric Exercise and the Cardiovascular System," *Modern Concepts of Cardiovascular Disease* (New York: American Heart Association, New York), March 1972, pp. 11-15.
16. *Ibid.*
17. DETRY, J. M., *Exercise Testing and Training in Coronary Heart Disease* (Baltimore, Maryland: Williams & Wilkins, 1973), pp. 57-59.
18. KAVANAGH, T., SHEPHARD, R. H., and PANDIT, V., "Marathon Running after Myocardial Infarction." *J A M A*, September 16, 1974, pp. 1602-1605.

7

assessments for phase II cardiac rehabilitation

Behavioral Objectives

After completion of this chapter, the reader should be able to:

■ describe six factors that influence a patient's willingness and ability to learn.

■ conduct a dialogue designed to effectively solicit health information from a patient.

■ use appropriate methods to control a nurse-patient conversation.

■ explain the purpose and components of the daily "mini assessments" performed by the nurse on Phase II patients.

■ name the three types of breath sounds and illustrate where they are heard on the chest.

Introduction

The second segment of an inpatient cardiac rehab program, Phase II, commences with transfer from the acute care unit to the progressive unit. Since physical location remains under the same roof, and since with increasing frequency, the same nursing staff covers both patient care areas, nursing care generally continues without major interruption. Nursing efforts during Phase II concentrate on patient-family education and gradual activity progression, each requiring initial and ongoing assessment for effective rehab planning.

The Educational Base

"The patient has the right to obtain from his physician complete current information concerning his diagnosis, treatment, and prognosis in terms the patient can be reasonably expected to understand."[1] The Patient's Bill of Rights publicly identifies the physician's responsibility. Equally important, the Standards of Nursing Practice set forth by the Congress for Nursing Practice explicity state the educational responsibilities of professional nurses.[2]

The Patient's Learning Status

The patient in Phase II has frequently entered a period of awareness of his health situation and, it is hoped, developed an acceptance of the diagnosis. Such a patient is ready for information concerning his problem and the alternatives available to him to deal with it.

Many factors influence the way information is presented by the nurse, the way information is received by the patient, and the eventual outcome of health teaching. Such things as physical and psychological readiness to learn, socioeconomic factors, past experiences, personal strengths and weaknesses, culture, motivation, and present level of understanding will all have direct bearing on presentation and receptivity. The more complete the nurse's profile of these factors in the patient's life, the better she will be able to meet his educational needs.

Sources of this information include the patient, family members, patient chart, physician and other health care members, and frequently the patient's colleagues or best friend. The nurse may choose to assemble the information via a deliberate interview, but more often the information is acquired less formally over a period of a few days by discussions with the patient and his family. Ideally, nurse-family rapport will have been established in Phase I and much information about learning status will have been acquired before the patient enters Phase II. Such information should be documented as it is gathered to form the assessment base for the Phase II teaching plan.

Physical and Psychological Influences. Patients who are psychologically distraught, who are experiencing feelings of hopelessness, or who are actively denying their sick status are not yet ready to learn about their health problem and its management. Such patients need continued emotional support and should be offered only information likely to help allay their anxieties and promote realistic acceptance.

Patients who are physically depleted, strongly sedated, or easily fatigued will find it difficult to concentrate or to expend the energy to learn. In such instances, the approach may be to delay teaching, to plan teaching in mini doses, or perhaps an alteration in the drug regimen would be appropriate. The nurse educator must be constantly alert to patient receptivity and modify the educational planning appropriately to meet needs and abilities.

As stated previously, the Phase II patient is usually in a period of awareness, the anxiety and/or denial generally having dissipated by about day three in CCU. The typical Phase II patient will be eager to begin acquiring information about the cause and course of his myocardial infarction and its treatment.

Socioeconomic Factors. The individual's ability to "afford" the illness, either emotionally or economically, can affect his preception of the illness and its importance. Patients who are economically deprived need to have their treatment plan proposed in such a way that they will be able to accept it. This may mean obtaining assistance through other professionals, the social service department, or community agencies for such things as helping the patient to procure his medications without undue financial hardship, providing an exercise program that is within his financial means, or helping him to formulate eating plans comprised of foods which are affordable to him yet within the guidelines of his prescribed diet.

The male patient in particular may find it emotionally unacceptable or uncomfortable to pursue a prescribed treatment plan due to feelings of decreased productivity or masculinity associated with the cardiac event. He may feel that he will be ineffective in the business world if he modifies his approach to work by endeavoring to reduce stresses and planning work in a more healthful manner. He may perceive the cardiac event as a very real threat to his economic livelihood and job stability (as well it may be) and, thus, in an effort to protect himself, find it easier to resist internalization of health information and never attempt behavioral change.

Reaction to the illness relative to his place in the family structure may also contribute to the patient's ability or inability to accept the cardiac event as fact and, thus, to be amenable to education. In a very dependent family structure, the patient may subconciously feel that if he accepts his illness and its inherent life changes, he will not be able to continue to provide within the expectations or needs of the other family members. Often the patient's behavior is affected as much by the reactions of the family members to his illness as by any other aspect of his illness.

Past Experiences. The adult patient has had a life of experiences which may either help or hinder his willingness to accept illness and to actively participate in planned education. Patients who have had satisfactory experiences with health professionals are likely to be more open to suggestions and teachings than patients with no previous experiences or those whose experiences have been unsatisfactory. Adults have much to contribute to the learning process because of past experiences and developed skills. They should be included as active participants with their ideas, attitudes, and skills being a valuable part of the process. Approaching the patient as an immature, dependent learner indicates that the nurse is an inexperienced or insecure teacher.

Personal Strengths and Weaknesses. Some patients will have already experienced the need to make behavioral changes in their life and have developed skills and attitudes effective in handling change. This valuable internal resource can be called upon as patients make life choices to implement other behavioral changes. Conversely, others find that throughout their life they are unable to actualize lasting behavioral changes. These patients will need added help and support in developing skills and attitudes necessary to make current desired changes.

Some patients derive strength from internal sources such as their life philosophy or religious beliefs. Others may find their main source of strength in family, close friends, or confidantes.

The nurse educator should strive to identify for each patient persons, aspects of personality, or past experiences from which he draws support and strength. Once identified, these strengths can be incorporated into the educational plan. Sources of weakness or detrimental influences should also be determined and efforts to alleviate or modify them initiated.

Culture. The patient's ethnic group or society, its language, attitude, skills, value systems, and shared judgments make up a valuable part of his personality and life. Nurses who work with particular ethnic groups should strive to understand their cultural traits in order to be more effective educators. Behavior modification suggestions must be made in line with established customs and ways of life.

Language barriers may pose a significant problem in communication between the patient and educator. In some instances, an interpreter or a bilingual professional with the patient's language skills may be needed to assist the primary educator. Family members may be the most helpful teaching intermediaries.

Motivation. The most important variable controlling the amount of learning that will occur is the patient's own motivation. He must feel that it is important to him to learn and believe that the information offered is necessary to his welfare.

Learning involves emotion and is most effective when there is a slight amount of anxiety present. For example, if the cardiac patient feels convinced that the pain he suffered was related to his heart, the anxiety of preventing recurrence will help motivate him to learn about the cause, treatment, and prevention of heart attacks. The adult patient who will learn most effectively will be the one with a strong intrinsic motivation to acquire the knowledge necessary to help him deal with his problem.

Figure 7-1 presents a graphic display of the influences reviewed above.

The Patient's Educational Needs

Some of the educational needs of the patient are dictated by the event itself while others are determined by the patient's life-style. A postmyocardial infarction patient may have any combination of educational needs. Fortunately, for patient and nurse educator alike, few patients ever have all anticipated educational needs. The nurse educator is responsible for assessing which

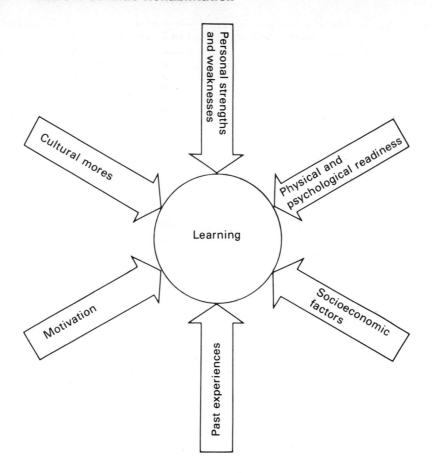

Figure 7-1. Learning influences.

educational needs pertain to each patient, as well as what factors may influence the educational process (discussed in the preceding section). Figure 7-2 presents an overview of Phase II educational needs.

Determination of the patient's current knowledge level in each educational area is part of the overall educational assessment. Health knowledge already possessed by the patient may be extensive or limited and may be correct or erroneous. The teaching plan constructed should carry the patient from his present level of knowledge to the point where he will be able to effect a behavioral change in his life.

Soliciting Information. Educational assessment depends upon effective nurse-patient communication. Attention to question structure and techniques of controlling a discussion—good communication methods—is essential to a good understanding of the patient's knowledge. The following is a basic review of

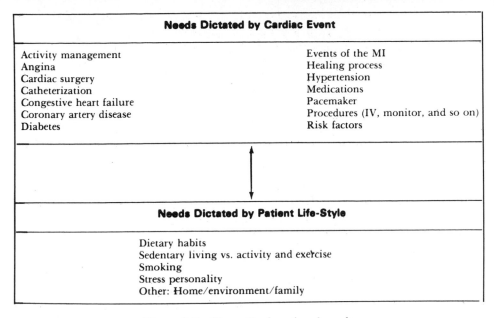

Figure 7-2. Phase II educational needs.

some types of questions and communication techniques that may be helpful to the nurse as she conducts a formal interview or has a spontaneous discussion with a patient.

Open-ended Question. An open-ended question is one that requires a statement or description for an answer. It cannot be answered with a simple yes or no. Questions that begin with what, where, why, or how are open-ended. For example, "What do you understand about your heart attack?" (Assuming, of course, that the patient has previously described his problem as a heart attack!) "What medications do you take each day?" "How do you take your nitroglycerin?" "When do you take it?" "Why do you think it helps your chest pain?" And so on.

Closed Question. The closed question can be answered with yes or no. It can be very useful, particularly for clarifying information already given by the patient ("Did you need to use nitroglycerin today?") or for simple information ("Have you seen this brochure before?"). The closed question, if used at the wrong time, can provide misinformation for the educator. Consider the following example: A patient has been experiencing chest discomfort with activity for which nitroglycerin, p.r.n. has been prescribed. He has taken a nitroglycerin tablet on six occasions and each time it has failed to relieve his discomfort.

Closed Question: "Do you know how to take your nitroglycerin?"
Answer: "Yes." (Thinking: Everyone knows how to take a pill!!)
Open-ended Question: "How do you take your nitroglycerin?"
Answer: "Usually with water." (The patient's misconception has been identified.)

Leading Question. Some questions imply the answer you would like to receive, and most patients are inclined to follow the lead and try to tell you what you want to hear. Example: "You do understand about how to use your nitroglycerin, don't you?"

Checklist Question. This type of question asks for multiple choice answers and can become very confusing. For example, "If you were to take a nitroglycerin for chest discomfort and it didn't work, do you think you should try another one, try taking two at the same time, or try aspirin instead?" By the time the question has been asked, the patient has either forgotten the question, gotten lost in the answers, or has fallen asleep. Checklist questions are not recommended for nurse-patient communication.

Techniques for Controlling Communication. Using *silence* as a technique is to use as little control over the conversation as possible. This is a good technique to use initially in determining the amount of information a patient may have on a given topic. Just ask, with an open ended question, "What have you learned about your nitroglycerin and how to use it?" and then silently listen. Listening attentively and hearing what is said is a skill worth cultivating. Listening and use of silence are not passive on the part of the nurse. Body language and facial expression convey interest and are an encouragement for the patient to continue.

Sometimes there is a lull in the conversation, a period of silence on the part of the patient. Perhaps the patient needs this second of quiet to formulate a way of expressing a thought or to decide whether or not to relate another fact. It is best, if you sense this may be the case, to let the silence stand and not interrupt with a comment or another question.

Facilitation is a technique by which communication is encouraged by something said or an action performed. Facilitating techniques should not specify the information wanted or direct the conversation to a specific area.

Active body language which facilitates conversation includes nodding the head, a quizzical look, smiling at a particular statement or laughing appropriately, frowning as the patient describes something which is displeasing to him, and so on. It is body language which says, in effect, I understand how you feel, I'm with you.

Another facilitating technique is to repeat the last few words of one of the patient's statements, but in a questioning tone. For example, "The nitroglycerin didn't have *any* effect on your pain?" This technique suggests that the listener would like the information expanded, but the decision to do so is voluntary on the part of the speaker.

Often in talking with patients, observation of behavior leads to belief that the patient is experiencing certain emotions not supported by his conversation. *Confrontation* is a response to the patient's nonverbal communication. It should be done in the form of a statement of observation made not as an accusation: "You seem nervous this afternoon." Not, "Why are you nervous this afternoon?" The patient's response might be, "I developed a rash on the back of my legs and it is hard for me to sit still for very long. I guess you thought I was nervous because I'm squirming around in my chair."

Confrontation should not be overused. Patients do not enjoy being made to feel that their every action is being scrutinized. But occasionally, confrontation is an effective technique, frequently bringing the conversation to an entirely new topic that otherwise would be missed.

Documenting Educational Assessments

Results of the educational assessment may be summarized within the progressive unit admission/transfer note if most information is available initially, or educational status notations can be entered in conjunction with other nursing assessments on a daily basis. Exact methods of charting will depend upon the record system used by the hospital. The record should include statement of the educational needs which have been identified, the present level of understanding regarding those needs, factors which will influence the education (psychological, environmental, and so on), and patient strengths and weaknesses (see Table 7-1 for an example).

Assessing Activity Readiness

Transfer from the acute unit implies that the patient's physical condition is stable. His cardiac diagnosis, however, implies potentiality for cardiac change and possibly crises. Assuring stability of the patient's physical state prior to advancing activities is the responsibility of the nurse specialist in Phase II.

Initial Assessment

If the Phase II nurse specialist is seeing the patient for the first time, the standard approach of taking a nursing history (See Chapter 12) complemented by a cardiovascular examination (See Chapter 17) and a pulmonary examination (see below) is best for getting acquainted. If the nurse has already worked with the patient in Phase I, an abbreviated history and physical examination to update nursing information may be all that is needed. Information noted about the patient's physical state becomes the reference to which changes are compared as the patient recovers.

Mini Assessment

Activities in Phase II are designed to gradually require increases in energy output. Physical signs are used to gauge tolerance/intolerance to each increase (See Chapter 3). The nurse specialist precedes each activity increase with a "mini" physical assessment. Each mini workup usually includes auscultation of the heart and lungs, apical heart rate, blood pressure, and a brief questioning period to uncover any new symptoms the patient may have experienced. This evaluation is aimed at uncovering new or developing problems that may contraindicate the planned activity.

Table 7-1

Documentation of Phase II Educational Assessment

Multiple learning needs may be documented in categories as shown or in a summary paragraph.

Educational Needs	Level of Learning	Influencing Factors
CAD	"Blockage of blood vessel to heart muscle by fats collecting inside the artery."	Retained what was taught in CCU.
Events of MI	"Muscle died from lack of blood and a scar will form in that area."	Realistic outlook.
Angina	"Small heart attacks."	No previous awareness of angina.
Risk factors	"It runs in the family."	Father died of second MI.
Medications	"I don't know what they have been giving me."	Trust of health professionals without questioning.
Smoking	"They say it's bad for my heart, but I don't know why; can understand about it being bad for lungs."	Both wife and son smoke.
Stress	"You gotta work hard to get ahead."	Recently retired from steel mill.
Sedentary living	"Now that I'm retired, I try to take life easy."	Work was only physical activity.
Diet	"My wife takes care of that."	Ethnic heritage, most cooking in family tradition.
Home activities	"Nurse says I'm supposed to be active up to a point, but my Dad didn't do much after his heart attack."	Negative past experience.

Pulmonary Assessment

Pulmonary complications are among the deconditioning effects of bed rest. Many cardiac patients have concomitant pulmonary disease. Phase II physical assessments, therefore, should include nursing evaluation of pulmonary status. The following review of major pulmonary assessments is offered to stress the fact that abnormal findings in this system, most likely to be uncovered during early hospitalization, may directly affect Phase II activity planning.

Breathing Patterns. The pattern of the patient's breathing can be observed while inspecting the patient's chest. Abnormal patterns familiar to the nurse specialist are reviewed in Table 7-2.

Table 7-2
Abnormal Breathing Patterns

Name	Description	Associations
Dyspnea	Difficulty in breathing	Emphysema, acute cardiac disease, pulmonary embolism
Tachypnea	Abnormal rapid breathing	Hysteria syndrome, nervousness
Hyperpnea	Abnormal deep and rapid respirations	Pain, febrile or cardiac disease, hysteria
Cheyne-Stokes	Periods of hyperpnea alternating with periods of apnea in a repeating cycle of gradually increasing and decreasing rate and depth of respiration	Heart failure, cerebral disease, drug sensitivities
Orthopnea	Dyspnea in the recumbent position	Asthma, emphysema, heart failure
Paroxysmal nocturnal dyspnea	Sudden dyspnea which occurs at night and awakens patient	Heart failure

Normal Breath Sounds. To effectively auscultate the lungs, the nurse must be familiar with normal breath sounds.

Vesicular Sounds. Air moving through the bronchioles and alveoli causes turbulence as it is distributed to the individual alveoli. The resulting sound is called vesicular breathing. Vesicular sounds are the normal sounds heard over most of the chest surface.

Bronchovesicular Sounds. Bronchovesicular sounds are caused by a mixture of vesicular sounds and the sound produced as air travels in an out through the tracheobronchial tree. Bronchovesicular sounds are best heard where the

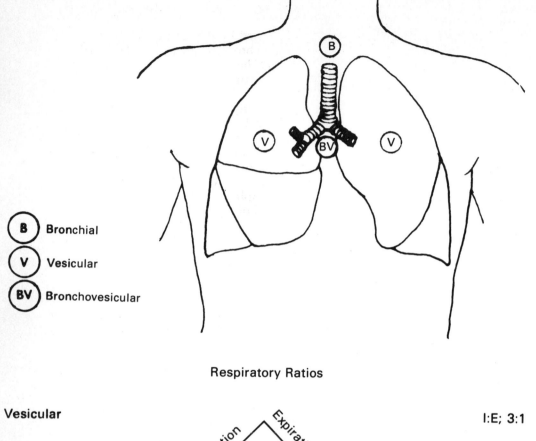

Figure 7-3.   Areas for auscultation of normal breath sounds.

tracheobronchial tree is close to the chest surface. If bronchovesicular sounds are heard over the main portion of the lung, it may indicate pulmonary consolidation.

Bronchial Sounds. Bronchial sounds are caused by the vibration of air as it travels through the trachea and two main stem bronchi and are heard normally over the trachea and two main stem bronchi. If heard over the lung tissue, such sounds would indicate a condition in which the lung tissue is compressed, such as pleural effusion or pneumonia.

Figure 7-3 illustrates areas for auscultating breath sounds. Length of inspiration and expiration as heard with each sound is also diagrammed. Inspiration/expiration ratios are useful in distinguishing sounds. **Adventitious Sounds.** Sounds heard in addition to the normal breath sounds just reviewed are called adventitious sounds. Caused by secretions and exudate, rhonchi and râles are the major types.

Use of these terms varies somewhat geographically and each nurse should be familiar with the usage of her coworkers and physicians. Table 7-3 presents a summary description of abnormal sounds.

Table 7-3
Adventitious Sounds

Name	Description	Associations
Rhonchi Coarse (sonorous) Sibilant	Vibrations of mucous strands in larger bronchi and trachea	Bronchitis Asthma Emphysema Bronchiectasis
Râles Fine Medium Coarse	Produced when an excess of fluid accumulates in the alveoli or any portion of the tracheobronchial tree	Pneumonia Congestive heart failure Pulmonary edema Bronchitis Pulmonary congestion

Summary

Results of Phase II assessments, both educational and physical, are summarized as patient problems/needs to begin the written rehab plan. Nursing consideration is next given to how to help the patient solve his problems and meet his needs.

(Patient ID Stamp)		
	C. P.	**CARDIAC REHAB PROGRESS NOTES**

Date/Time	PROGRESS NOTES
5/5/XX 2 p.m.	Transferred to PCCU:
	S. Seems relieved to be out of CCU. "Now maybe I'll get some exercise so I can get out of here." More freely asking questions about capabilities after discharge. Anxious to know more. Eager to involve his wife in discussions.
	O. Reviewed Phase I records. Physical condition has been stable since admission. Early activities were tolerated well. Will pursue fear of death problem remaining. Educationally, seems to understand MI and healing. Relationship of personal risk factors needs to be established and possible modifications discussed. Influences on educational planning: well educated, close family relationship, lives on a farm, used to being self-sufficient and hard working, works full time as teacher plus farming, negative experience of brother dying of AMI 2 years ago.
	A. Willing and able to begin Phase II rehab.
	P. Current needs and problems summarized on Rehab Plan. Objectives reviewed with patient, agreeable and anxious to begin.
	n.d. R.n.

References

1. AMERICAN HOSPITAL ASSOCIATION, *A Patient's Bill of Rights* (Chicago, Illinois: American Hospital Association, 1973).
2. CONGRESS for NURSING PRACTICE, *Standards of Nursing Practice* (Kansas City, Missouri: American Nurses' Association, 1973).

8

planning of phase II cardiac rehabilitation

Behavioral Objectives

After completion of this chapter, the reader should be able to:

- identify common nursing goals of Phase II.
- recommend activities appropriate to Phase II and suggest a structured approach for implementation.
- discuss the need for sexual expression during hospitalization.
- name and explain the domains and the stages of learning.
- define behavioral objective and discuss use of objectives in patient education.
- construct an educational plan for a given cardiac rehab topic.
- select appropriate teaching methods for each of the domains of learning.
- identify resources for cardiac teaching aids.

Introduction

Upon entering Phase II, the acute myocardial infarction patient may be out of immediate life-threatening danger, but continued recovery and eventual optimal health depend upon effective planning of health care for the remainder of hospitalization. Meeting rehab needs and solving health problems are of mutual concern to patient and nurse.

Since many postmyocardial infarction patients share certain problems and concerns, some rehab needs can be anticipated and planned for in advance. Planning starts with goal setting. Table 8-1 lists common nursing goals of Phase II.

Table 8-1
Common Nursing Goals of Phase II Cardiac Rehabilitation

Physiological	To further minimize the negative effects of prolonged inactivity and to assist the patient to gradually resume activities of daily living through a graduated activity program
Psychosocial	To continue to provide support to the patient and significant others and to offer assistance to ease necessary adjustments
Educational	To provide the patient and significant others with:
	The knowledge needed to understand and effect changes in life-style.
	The skills needed to accomplish change.
	The attitude and motivation to sustain change.

Planning to Meet Physiological Goals

By the time most myocardial infarction patients are transferred to the intermediate unit, they are ready, willing, and able to increase their activity.

Selecting Activities

Activities in which patients participate during Phase II are a continuation of those started in Phase I, emphasizing daily activities to enable self-care upon discharge. Patients in Phase II spend most of their day out of bed in a chair and walking in the hospital corridors. In some programs, progressive activity is carried out in the physical therapy department; while in others, it is done at the bedside. Table 8-2 lists activities appropriate for Phase II.

Stair climbing prior to discharge is the climax of Phase II activities. Patients need to be given the assurance that they are capable of performing this familiar activity upon going home. Carrying out the stair execution in the hospital under monitored conditions provides the assurance of knowing the activity is "safe."

Table 8-2
Activities for Phase II Rehabilitation

Self-Care Activities	Self-dressing, feeding, and personal hygiene Bathroom privileges, including bathing in tub, shaving at sink, and so on
Physical Activities	Sitting in a chair, supporting feet and arms with chair back high enough to allow head resting Active range of motion of all extremities Trunk bending and twisting at moderate speed and degree of stretch Walking in hospital corridor, increasing distance each day Stair climbing prior to discharge
Occupational Activities	Work reduction techniques for everyday activities and certain occupations: Cooking and serving a meal Arranging work tools and equipment Lifting and carrying Good body mechanics
Craft Activities	Selection should reduce isometric involvement, limit preparation and clean-up time, and be of interest: Copper tooling, leather craft Knitting, crocheting, needlepoint Sketching, painting Model building

Preferably, the patient will have the opportunity to perform stair climbing several times prior to discharge. This one activity does much to reduce anxieties about things which traditionally have been taboo for cardiac patients.

Depending on the physical layout of the hospital, stair climbing may be performed in any of the following ways:

- Descend a flight of stairs and return by elevator.
- Ascend one-half flight of stairs, rest, and then descend.
- Ascend a flight of stairs and return by elevator.
- Perform equivalent climbing work on steps in the physical therapy department.

Activity guidelines are the same for Phase II as used to guide activities in Phase I (See Chapter 3). Assessment of the patient's activity tolerance is an ongoing nursing responsibility.

Structuring Progression

Progressive activity programs incorporate the type of activities just described in a gradual manner beginning with those requiring the least energy and progressing. For convenience, activities grouped by MET categories may be prelisted in steps or levels.[1] In constructing a progression, the number of steps may be arranged to correspond to the average number of days in the progressive unit (or in the hospital if step 1 begins in the CCU). Figure 8-1 presents a sample Phase II activity progression. Progression is carried out according to the physician's order and patient tolerance.

Planning to Meet Psychosocial Goals

The fact that the patient is in a less restricted environment, that he is participating in an increasing number of activities, and that plans are being made for discharge is a psychological boost to both patient and family in Phase II. Continued support and reassurance will be needed to maintain and strengthen this new found optimism.

A well-informed spouse can be a tremendous asset to the patient during the remaining hospitalization and the spouse's participation in rehab planning should be invited. Private nurse-spouse discussions, bedside conferences, and group conferences can all help the spouse to help the patient.

Sexual expression should be encouraged in Phase II. The spouse should understand that sex encompasses more than the "sexual act" and that at this time, it is common for cardiac patients to have sexual needs. Love and its inherent sexuality may be demonstrated in a number of ways that are safe and acceptable to the patient's level of health. Touching—holding hands, a caress, a kiss—and open communication help the patient retain his sexuality and self-esteem.

The spouse should also understand that it is quite normal for a patient to go through a period of depression and grief which may have begun while in the CCU and may continue or recur in later hospitalization. During this time, patients frequently have little desire to be sexually active and may even experience secondary impotence. The spouse plays an important role in helping to counteract this depression and the increase in physical activity also helps demonstrate to the patient that "all is not lost." If the spouse is given a clear understanding of this process, interpretation of reactions as sexual rejection will be less likely.

Some male patients, in an attempt to prove their continued masculinity, will exhibit overt sexual behavior to female nurses. They may flirt with the nurses, use objectional language, tell provocative jokes, and become sexually aggressive. Such individuals usually respond to being confronted with their behavior in a kind manner. The nurse may question the patient about his realization of how often he refers to sex. Her attitude should convey her liking of and respect for the patient as a person. Confrontation provides an opportune time to discuss the patient's feelings of himself as a sexual being and to provide him with needed information. Helping the patient become aware that sexual

Figure 8-1. Recommended Phase II activities (2-3 METs).

Level	1	2	3	4	5	6	7	8	9	10
Continue activities as in CCU										
Sit in chair for meals	Breakfast & dinner	All meals								
Ambulate in room as desired										
Hall ambulation		Once a day	Twice a day	As desired						
Group education classes			PRN							
Bathroom privileges	For BM	For BM	PRN							
Tub bathing										
Active body stretch and flexibility movements					Once a day	Twice a day	Three times a day			
Down one flight stairs										
Up one flight stairs										
Up and down one flight stairs										
Predischarge exercise test										

☐ Not Appropriate   ☐ Appropriate

86

dysfunction is not the norm after a cardiac event and answering questions he may have at this time may be achieved during general conversation with the patient. Discussion of sexual activity should be handled in the same manner as any other activity. For example, the nurse might say, "You may have been wondering what you will be capable of doing now that you have had a heart attack. Most patients are able to return to their normal activities and participate in things they enjoyed prior to the event, like driving, dancing, sexual activity, golf, jogging, and so on. Some of these activities may have to be resumed slowly at first, but soon can be enjoyed at their previous level."

More information may be offered at this time if the patient seems receptive. Such a statement conveys to the patient the nurse's willingness to discuss the subject of sex and the important fact that he may expect to enjoy sexual activity in the future.

The spouse may be more ready to discuss sexual activity once she feels the immediate danger to life has passed. A one-to-one conference affords the opportunity to discuss the psychological implications of a myocardial infarction and the spouse's role in helping the patient maintain his masculinity.

Planning to Meet Educational Goals

Assessment of a patient's educational needs and the factors influencing his receptivity to education was presented in Chapter 7. Once learning problems are identified, planning educational solutions begins. Knowing what to teach is the easiest part of educational planning. Knowing how to teach is the most important capability of the Phase II nurse specialist.

Process of Adult Learning

Effective learning, that which results in a desired change, usually involves all three areas of human behavior to some degree. The *cognitive domain* deals with mental processes, knowledge, intellectual abilities, and understanding. The *affective domain* involves attitudes, feelings, and emotions. The *psychomotor domain* pertains to voluntary physical movement.

The patient who has been able to correctly manage a prescribed dietary regimen, for example, will have an understanding of the diet's relationship to his disease and the components and methods of its management (cognitive domain), the desire or attitude necessary to plan adherence (affective domain), and the physical ability to prepare and ingest food (psychomotor domain).
Stages of Learning. Patients progress through a series of developmental stages or learning levels in pursuit of desired behavioral change. On a given level, needs may be mainly cognitive, affective, or psychomotor.
Awareness. In the first stage, the patient becomes aware of his health problem. For the cardiac patient, this involves confirmation of the fact that the discomfort he experienced was related to his heart and not to a less threatening body system. During this stage, the patient needs not only the cognitive information about what has happened, but also assistance in dealing with the information emotionally in order to develop the desired affect whereby he will be able to finally say to himself, "I can accept the fact and I do believe that I have suffered a heart attack."

Table 8-3
Learning Process of the Cardiac Patient

Problem Awareness	Acquisition of Information	Management Plan
Psychological state Anxiety/denial	**Psychological state** Awareness →	**Psychological state** Resolution →
Educational Needs Cognitive Description of the problem, diagnoses and information for development of a mental image of the problem	**Educational Needs** Cognitive Process of an MI Anatomy Physiology Healing process Risk factors Patient self-role in treatment plan Risk factor identification and modification Implementation of prescribed diet Exercise Medication and so on	**Educational Needs** Cognitive Discussion of personal health objectives Practical ideas for methods of attainment within usual environment and relationships
Affective Support in accepting the diagnoses	Affective Personal risk factors and self-benefits of modifying risk factors Receive support, reassurance and ideas from others who have been able to modify their risk factors	Affective Group and individual support in persisting with plan Continued motivation Satisfactory experiences and rewards of praise and encouragement
	Psychomotor Self-pulse monitoring techniques Self-medication techniques Dietary management techniques (choosing appropriate foods from hospital menu) Smoking cessation techniques Stress reduction techniques	Psychomotor Attainment of skills resulting in performance of desired behavior

As reviewed in Chapter 3, the patient in Phase I is typically the patient who needs to become aware of his problem. Some patients progress through this level of learning rather rapidly, being able to accept the diagnosis while others may remain at a standstill. The patient who convinces himself that the source of discomfort experienced was not his heart or that the medical staff has made an error in diagnosis is not likely to learn. In some cases, where the diagnosis is not clear cut and the patient is left with the explanation that it may or may not have been his heart, it is difficult for the patient to progress to a higher level of learning.

Acquisition of Knowledge. The second stage of learning involves acquiring information and knowledge about the problem. Patients try to discover what alternatives are available. At this level, they are ready for an explanation of coronary artery disease, risk factors and their influence on coronary artery disease, and alternatives that are available to them in their proposed treatment plan. This type of knowledge is important in meeting the cognitive domain of learning. Patients in this stage also have an acute need for assistance in developing an appropriate affect toward the treatment of their disease.

Group discussions among patients can be a very effective method of providing support and encouragement. Examples of others' experiences are helpful in developing affect. The accumulation and internalization of knowledge, the development of motor skills necessary to utilize the knowledge (as in learning to count one's pulse), and the adoption of an appropriate attitude are all important components of the second stage of learning.

Action. In the third stage of learning, the patient actually begins to institute the behavioral change. He tries to develop a means by which he will be able to incorporate the knowledge, attitudes, and skills to which he has been exposed into his own life situation. Again, there is a need for cognitive information, as in personalizing the general knowledge and principles to his environment and abilities. There is also the affective component in that he must persist with the attitude of trying the behavioral change and develop a means by which he can be comfortable with the changes among his family and peers. This may involve changing the affect of some of the family members. For example, creating an understanding in the family members that the patient's low-cholesterol diet is just as beneficial for them as it is for the patient would help them to develop a cooperative attitude in implementing the diet as the family food plan.

The third stage of learning usually involves a greater amount of utilization of the psychomotor domain. This is the stage in which the patient is actually endeavoring to perform the desired behavior. The educator must know the patient's neuromuscular capabilities and make alterations in the educational plan in the event that the patient has a problem with skills needed. Table 8-3 summarizes the learning process.

Behavioral Objectives

"Behavioral objectives are statements that describe the behavior the student is expected to exhibit as a result of one or more learning experiences."[2] Objectives serve as both planning and evaluation tools.

Formulating objectives is the first step in planning education. Many useful approaches to writing objectives have been recommended.[3-5] One practical method is to construct the statement in two parts:

- the goal statement to specify the change in behavior desired of the learner.
- the time criteria to express when the behavior will be evaluated.

Use of this type of objective provides the advantage of preparing in advance and storing a battery of goal statements for each of the anticipated cardiac educational topics. Time criteria, more likely to vary from patient to patient based on individual abilities and expectations, can be added to finalize objectives.

Each educational topic may have a number of behavioral objectives. Using smoking as an example, the ultimate goal is for the patient to understand why smoking is harmful to his health and to stop smoking. To accomplish this goal, most patients need to

- know what effects smoking has on the body (cognitive).
- have the desire to stop smoking (affective).
- stop smoking (psychomotor).

Using the approach just described for preparing behavioral objectives, the goals for the smoking patient can be translated as follows:

- Patient will state three effects smoking has on his cardiovascular system before discharge.
- Patient will state his intention to stop smoking and set a date to initiate action before discharge.
- Patient will abstain from use of tobacco upon return to home.

Now the objectives are specific. They give good direction to what will need to be taught and are a guide for establishing an educational plan. The same objectives also provide a means by which to evaluate patient outcomes.

Other educational topics may require many objectives to assure that the patient is able to live his treatment plan. Dietary teaching, for example, would need objectives to determine that the patient has an understanding of the relationship between the disease and the diet, the foods which are allowed/not allowed, balanced meal planning, choosing the correct products by reading the labels, what to do when eating out, food preparation, and so on.

Setting objectives is not an exclusive function of the nurse educator. Remembering that the patient is an equal partner in his health planning, the nurse's role is to help the patient understand the problems that have been identified, their impact on the patient's health, the options available for dealing with the problems, and the potential consequences of accepting status quo. The patient's role, given the preceding information, is to help set his own health goals indicated via behavioral objectives. The patient and nurse educator should discuss health goals, with the patient expressing changes he perceives as important and the nurse recommending certain changes in the patient's health interest. The end result of such a planning session should be mutually agreeable health goals documented as behavioral objectives.

Caution: not every patient is going to stop smoking because a nurse lists smoking cessation as a priority objective. As difficult as it may be to accept at times, the Phase II nurse specialist in an educator role must realize that the patient has the right to make the decisions to continue life habits which may be injurious to his health. It is his health and his life. As stated previously, nursing responsibility is to furnish the patient with enough information to allow him to make a knowledgeable choice.

Most patients realize that smoking is a major coronary risk factor, but may not know the effect smoking has on their hearts, arteries, and red blood cells. If after initial discussion, a patient is determined to continue smoking, he should be provided with factual information of the effects of smoking on his body and asked to re-evaluate his attitude about continuing the habit. If he still intends to smoke, persistent objection by the nurse will be interpreted as nagging and will only serve to alienate the patient. Accept the patient's refusal and concentrate on other objectives more likely to be accomplished.

The Educational Plan

Once objectives have been formulated, an educational plan needs to be developed. The educational plan is a written outline that answers the following questions for a selected educational topic:

What factual information should be included in teaching this topic?
What means are available to present the information (pamphlets, flip charts, slides, films, and so on)?
What attitude will enhance understanding and acceptance of the information?
What can be done to stimulate development of the desired attitude?
What skills does the patient need to achieve the objectives?
What methods and materials can be used to teach necessary skills?

Once answers to the above questions are formulated, the choices of information, methods, and materials are organized into a sequential plan of education.

For example, drug education is a specific need of Phase II cardiac patients. Medication compliance may mean the difference between sickness and health, and medication education may mean compliance. In order to take their medications safely and effectively, patients need to have an understanding of their drug therapy in relation to their specific problem.

Patient education concerning drugs should begin early enough in the hospital stay to allow time for patient and family to absorb the information, feel comfortable with it, and have their understanding evaluated. Drug education for family members should encourage their active assistance with medication management after the patient's discharge with resulting increase in compliance. Table 8-4 outlines a sample plan for drug education.

Methods of Teaching

Teaching the Cognitive Domain. Information may be given by various methods, including group lecture, individual instruction, written materials, programmed learning materials, audiovisual aids, visual aids, tape recordings, charts, pictures, graphs, television, and so on. Any mode of education by which information is passed from one individual to another can be considered a method of meeting the cognitive domain of learning.

Table 8-4
Educational Plan for Medications

Patient Behavioral Objectives

Prior to discharge, the patient will be able to:
Name and visually identify each drug he is taking.
Explain in his own words, the effect of each drug on his condition.
Describe expected side effects and possible adverse reactions to each drug.

Cognitive Information

Teaching should include the following:
Name and description of each drug; patient should be told if a drug has more than one name, for example, Digoxin/Lanoxin; patient should be allowed to see and/or touch each drug to become familiar with it.
Explanation of the action of each drug specific to the patient's condition, for example, "Lasix—to help prevent the fluid accumulation which causes your heart to pump harder than necessary." "Coumadin—to make your blood thinner so it isn't as likely to clot and cause another heart attack; and it's easier for your heart to pump if the blood isn't quite so thick."

Explicit directions and/or demonstrations of proper administration of each drug; method should be specified, for example, oral, sublingual, chewing, and so on; times and circumstances should be specified, for example three times a day can mean (1) three times during waking hours (morning, midday, before bed), (2) three times equally spaced around the clock (7 a.m. - 3 p.m. - 11 p.m.), (3) with each meal. (Should it be before, during, or after eating?)
Explanation of precautions to be taken with each drug, for example, nitroglycerin should be stored in dark bottle; aspirin should not be taken while on Coumadin.
Explanation of expected side effects, for example, headache with nitroglycerin, and potential adverse reactions, such as skin rash, nausea and vomiting, diarrhea, and so on; patients should be advised to report these events to their physicians.

Methods and Aids

Methods effective in providing the information:
Small group sessions with patients on the same drugs.
One-to-one teaching (or nurse to family) may be used as or to supplement group sessions.
Aids to enhance learning:
Actual drugs
Flip chart with drug pictures and facts
Summary sheets or cards on each drug for the patient to keep for review and reference

---

The educator needs to have a clear understanding of the goals of a particular educational topic and the current level of understanding of the learner in relation to the topic before considering which method will most effectively reach desired cognition in the learner. Materials and methods should be designed to build a bridge of knowledge to carry the learner from his present level of understanding to the point where he will be able to meet his objectives.

Cognitive information should be offered on the level of the patient's ability to understand. For example, a poor reader might benefit from a pamphlet which presents the information in a cartoon or graphic fashion, a person with poor eyesight may be able to utilize pamphlets with oversized print, a person without previous medical experiences and a limited medical knowledge and vocabulary might understand the information best if it is presented with the use of a model and other pictures to help him form a mental image of the topic.

Any prepared source of information should be very carefully critiqued by the educator prior to its use. Ideas, attitudes, and information change as more is learned about cardiac disease and its management. Prepared material chosen should reflect the most recent and accurate information.

Lectures are usually highly structured and allow little or no opportunity for audience participation. Lectures are useful when it is necessary to address a large audience or at times when a topic is being presented which the audience has little or no previous knowledge of and, thus, is likely to have little input. If it is necessary to present information in a lecture form, it is recommended that the lecturer allow time at the end of the lecture to answer questions from the audience and make clarifications.

Teaching the Affective Domain. Motivating a patient and helping him develop desired attitudes are sometimes more difficult to accomplish than imparting cognitive understanding. Methods which may be employed include group sessions, behavior modification techniques, and role playing.

Sometimes patients do not develop desired affect because they have incorrect information about the problem. For example, if a patient's past experiences had indicated to him that the treatment of choice for a cardiac patient is complete bed rest for the first few weeks, he is not likely to exhibit a cooperative attitude about early ambulation. In this instance, however, if his cognitive information is corrected and updated, he may develop an affect which will permit him to become a willing participant in early ambulation. This is another example of the importance of identifying the patient's level of knowledge relating to the topic prior to instituting education.

Group dynamics can be an important and effective adjunct to helping develop desired affect. Group members with similar problems can make a patient feel less isolated, relate changes they may have experienced in their attitudes toward the problem and its treatment, and lend each other support, both in the emotional and in practical methods of handling problems.

Groups afford members the opportunity to serve as coinstructors, bolstering their own egos. Learners are generally more receptive to a person who has had personal experience with the problem and the coinstructor patient can be a real asset to the nurse educator.

Peer pressure is an effective aid for developing affect and motivation. The patient group is the ideal place for peer influences. Patients in a group seem to have a natural tendency to encourage other patients to consider life changes which are in their health's interest.

In Phase II, a group may consist of two patients who are roommates or a larger group of patients who are ambulatory or who may be transported to a meeting room. The nurse as group leader should consider the personalities, common problems, and common educational needs of the members. Additional thought should be given to what each patient either needs from the group or what he is likely to be able to contribute to the group. Ideally, groups will contain a balance of personalities, experiences, and needs which will benefit all participants.

Satisfaction motivates learning and this is the principle upon which some techniques of behavior modification are based. If we can provide a learner with a satisfying experience, he is likely to want to repeat that experience, having associated it with the feeling of satisfaction. Positive reinforcement is just as important to the adult learner as it is to a child. Positive reinforcement (praise) immediately following a desired behavior (such as adherence to dietary regimen) increases the probability that the behavior will be repeated.

Role playing can help the patient view his problem from a different perspective. He might, for example, role play his wife trying to convince him to decrease his workload and substitute more leisurely activities. He may role play the educator in the group situation which may lead to a firmer conviction in his own mind of the importance of the topic he was teaching. Using a subtle approach such as, "Yesterday we were having a good discussion on why you felt it was important to stop smoking. Why don't you share your thoughts with John?" will place the patient in the role-playing situation, yet not raise his anxieties unduly.

Teaching the Psychomotor Domain. Before initiating education pertaining to the psychomotor domain of learning, it is necessary to determine that the patient has the neuromuscular capability to perform the task. If it is found that he does not have the ability to perform, consideration must be given to what alterations or modifications are possible to meet the same objective via a different route. For example, your objective is that the patient be able to regulate his postdischarge walking program according to his heart rate response. The usual method for a heart rate check is for the patient to use a watch with a second hand and to count his radial pulse. Problem: this patient is unable to palpate his own radial pulse (although it is strong in each wrist). Therefore alternatives are necessary. Alternatives to the usual teaching method include the following:

Try the carotid pulse.
Try the temporal pulse.
Have the patient use a stethoscope and count the pulse apically.
Teach the patient's wife to take the pulse and have her accompany the patient on his walks.

The following is an example of teaching the common psychomotor task of pulse taking. (The prerequisite is the development of desired affect and knowledge.)

The patient must be given a good mental image of the task to be performed and have already acquired the cognitive information and developed the desire (affect) to perform the task. He should understand the "why" as well as the "how."

"The beating, or pulse, that you are feeling is caused by your heart pumping blood to your muscles. The more your muscles work, the more blood they need; the more blood needed, the more your heart has to work, and you will know it is working faster because your pulse will be faster. The idea is to work your muscles enough so they don't get weak, but at the same time not to work your heart too hard while it is still healing . . ." Continue discussion giving specific heart rate guidelines.

In explaining the how, it is important not to skip steps under the assumption that "everybody knows that." Proceed through each step in sequence, being alert to the patient response, answering questions as they arise. If equipment is involved in the demonstration, check for proper operation prior to starting. Be certain that all needed supplies are available.

Prior to demonstration, determine that the patient has a watch with a second hand—in working order, and that the patient has a neuromuscular system capable of performing the task.

Choice of Hands. "If you wear your watch on your left wrist, it is easiest to use your left hand to feel the pulse because you will be able to see your watch easily. The tips of your fingers are very sensitive so you can use the tips of your three middle fingers on the left hand to feel your pulse."

Landmarks. "Hold your right hand flat and notice the fleshy part of your thumb at the side of the palm of the hand. Down near the wrist you can feel the end of the bone leading up to the thumb. From here slide your three fingers down from the bone onto the wrist and you will feel a slight indentation between one of the arm bones and some tendons. You can usually feel the pulse in this groove."

Method of Palpating. "Touch very lightly and continue to slowly increase the pressure until you can feel the pulsations easily. Now, continue to increase the pressure, and you will find it is more difficult to feel the pulse because the increased pressure is pushing the artery closed so blood can't get through. When you take your pulse, then, you can vary the pressure you are applying 'til you find the point where it is easiest for you to count the pulse, remembering that too light or too heavy pressure will make it difficult or impossible to count it."

Counting. "When you have a good feel of the pulse, you can count the number of times your heart is beating by timing the pulsations with your watch. You don't have to wait for the second hand to get to 12 to start counting, just be sure to remember where you started and start at any of the 5 or 15 minute marks. Begin counting the pulsations as the second hand leaves the mark you have chosen and count each pulsation, stopping when the second hand returns to the starting point. While you are counting the pulse, be aware of the regularity . . ." (followed by appropriate discussion of irregularities as pertinent to the individual patient—atrial fibrillation will normally be irregular, patient prone to premature beats will need guidelines as to when to call his physician in the event they become too numerous as will patients on antiarrhythmic medications, and so on).

Variety and Emphasis. Education is more interesting for both patient and educator if the learning stimulus is varied. For example, the topic "coronary artery disease" might be handled in the following sequence:

- Brief introduction by the nurse and simple pamphlet given for the patient to read.
- Film strip on coronary artery disease.
- Group educational session led by nurse utilizing model heart for demonstration.
- Individual discussion between patient and nurse, evaluation of patient understanding by nurse, all patient questions answered.

Not only is the information more interesting if presented in a variety of ways, but the incorporation of teaching aids, in this instance literature, film strips, and heart model, stimulates more physical senses and promotes a higher degree of learning. People learn better by doing and participating actively in the learning process, and sensory stimulation increases the degree of active participation.

When we teach, much of what we say is directed toward developing desired affect while some of what we say is cognitive information which we want the patient to understand and remember. There are some techniques which, if properly employed, are useful in helping the patient sort significant points from support information:

- Visual aids which display the important points, handouts, pamphlets, diagrams, and so on.
- Planned repetition in the presentation of important words or phrases.
- Dynamic use of gestures or body language during discussion of the most pertinent information.
- Emphatic statements such as, The important thing to remember is . . . , Don't forget . . . , This part is especially important. . . .
- Topic summaries quickly reviewing the important points in order.

Throughout the teaching process, goals must be kept in sight. All that is taught should be relevant to the goal. The most important question that the educator must keep asking herself and the patient to assure that goals are being approached is *How is this going to work out for you when you get home?* The ultimate objective is for the patient to be able to live his rehab plan in his own environment. Many times, the Phase II patient is so busy learning and coping with today's problems that he has not actually thought ahead to how he will implement the desired behaviors and use new health information in his daily home life. It is all well and good, for example, if the patient is able to discuss the effects of smoking on his body and state the desire to stop, but what if he is returning home to a family of four, all of whom are heavy smokers? The real meaning of patient education is making it all work for the patient, sometimes an awesome challenge.

Teaching Aids

Visual aids to education are readily available and are frequently utilized by nurse educators. Sources to be contacted include drug companies, voluntary health agencies (American Heart Association, American Lung Association,

American Cancer Society), government agencies, and publishers. Some hospitals and private groups have published their own materials and may be willing to share or sell them. There is a wealth of printed material available in the form of leaflets, brochures, posters, and booklets.

Scale models of the heart are available from various companies. Plastic heart models may be purchased in hobby shops and assembled.

There are a number of audiovisual companies who are willing to demonstrate their viewing apparatus and films to nurses who are involved in patient education. Many hospitals or clinics have access to closed circuit television and have produced and videotaped special information programs for their cardiac patients.

Audio teaching aids in the form of cassette tapes or records, sometimes accompanied by a written script and/or illustrations, are useful in some instances. Strictly audio presentations should be of short duration because it is difficult to concentrate for long periods when only hearing is being stimulated. Whenever possible, visual materials should supplement audio materials.

Exhibitors attend seminars and offer participants the opportunity to become familiar with their products. This offers the nurse a chance to compare products, audiovisual programs, for example, and become more aware of what is available. Nursing journals and publishers' catalogues are another good source of information on materials available.

One source of teaching aids which is often overlooked is the educator's own creative ability to construct teaching aids. Artists sketch pads (wire bound type) make excellent flip charts that can be constructed for any teaching topic. For example:

- Exercise flip chart with pictures of different types of physical activities and exercise for instructing patients in do's and don'ts of exercise, allowable types, examples of isometric and isotonic activities.
- Diet flip chart with actual food labels, including the nutritional and ingredient section for discussion of consumer considerations, food choices, balanced meal planning, pictures of methods of food preparation, and so on.
- Drug flip chart with illustrations of and pertinent information on the most frequently used cardiac drugs (appropriate sections used to teach individual patients' prescribed medications).
- Topics which are difficult to explain, such as congestive heart failure; information arranged in a flip chart will help make it clear for the patient, as well as help the educator present it in an organized manner.

Word puzzles can be a fun teaching tool for patients who enjoy games. These may be constructed of words the patient should become familiar with in order to understand his problem, such as foods he should avoid, or on a more positive note, foods he may indulge in, or exercise and activity choices.

Nurses involved in patient education share ideas and information with each other, and nursing organization meetings can offer an excellent forum for such exchanges either formally or informally.

Summary

Even the most experienced nurse educator does not expect the postacute cardiac patient to change into a model of health overnight. Phase II is the beginning of acquiring new health information and modifying unhealthy habits. It will take time and practice for the new ways to become a comfortable and an enjoyable way of life for the patient. Participation in Phase III and Phase IV rehab programs as an outpatient will provide the means for additional education, encouragement, and guidance as the patient begins to live his rehab plan.

Table 8-5 summarizes the comprehensive educational process of Phase II.

Table 8-5
Cardiac Rehabilitation Education Summary

Nurse's Role	Patient's Role
Assessment	Awareness Level
Patient's educational needs	Assessment of problem and self in the situation
Patient's level of learning	
Patient's strengths and weaknesses	Assessment of personal risk factors
Planning	Acquisition Level
Plan for creating patient awareness of problem and needs	Consider options and make life choices
Patient behavioral objectives for each educational need	Identify personal behavioral objectives
Nurse and patient derive mutually agreeable behavioral objectives	
Implementation	Action Level
Support in problem acceptance	Participation in educational plan, gaining additional cognition, affect, and psychomotor skills while starting to live a rehab plan
Description of process of MI, risk factor influence	
Description of options available to deal with problem and risk factor reduction or modification	
Perform patient education in accordance with behavioral objectives	
Evaluation	Evaluation
Nurse and patient evaluate effects of education by determining if behavioral objectives have been met and assessing patient's attitude toward rehab continuation	

(Patient ID Stamp) C. P.			CARDIAC REHAB CARE PLAN	
Date Identified	**Need/Problem**	**Approach**	**Behavioral Objectives**	**Date Achieved Changed**
5/5/XX	**Physiological**		The patient will be able to	
	1. prevent decon- ditioning	1. } begin Phase II 2. } activity levels	1. } increase activity per- 2. } formance daily keeping	
			responses within estab- lished guidelines.	
	2. advance toward			
	level compatible with usual home activities			
	3. learn activity response assessment	3. a) teach patient how to take pulse	3. before discharge a) accurately count pulse at rest and during	
		b) teach patient his heart rate limit as	activity b) state his heart rate limit and describe in	
		activity guide	his own words the pur- pose of that limit	
	Psychosocial			
	4. unresolved fear of death from Phase I	4. encourage dis- cussion of remaining	4. indicate his realization that the immediate danger to life has passed through	
		fears; continue support	statements/actions concerning the future	

(Patient ID Stamp)				
	C. P.		**CARDIAC REHAB CARE PLAN**	
Date Identified	**Need/Problem**	**Approach**	**Behavioral Objectives**	**Date Achieved Changed**
			The patient will be able to	
	5. concern re	5. a) emphasize	5. before discharge	
	sufficient recovery by fall (4 months) to	necessity of one-step-at-a-time by	a) relate importance of gradual resumption of activities	
	resume full-time teaching *and* farming	teaching purposes of gradual	b) define isometric and isotonic exercise and give examples from his	
		increases b) teach "Types of Exercise"	usual daily activities and job	
		lesson to patient and wife		
	Educational			
	See #3 and#5			
	6. requesting diet guidelines	6. a) provide general information on low	6. before discharge a) explain the relationship between choles-	
		cholesterol diet	terol and heart disease b) express initial plans for dietary changes	
		b) arrange session with dietitian for		
		patient and wife		

(Patient ID Stamp) C. P.			CARDIAC REHAB CARE PLAN	
Date Identified	Need/Problem	Approach	Behavioral Objectives	Date Achieved Changed
	7. needs an in- creased aware- ness of effects of stress	7. discuss the nature of stress and physiological responses	The patient will be able to 7. begin to identify sources of stress in his life	
	8. medications: Valium 5 mg. t.i.d. NTG 1/100 gr. p.r.n.	8. a) discuss pur- pose of Valium during early recovery b) teach "Nitro- glycerin" lesson	8. before discharge a) relate the name, dose, purpose, and common side effects of dis- charge meds, and the times when each is to be taken b) for NTG also explain storage precautions and appropriate p.r.n. use	

(Patient ID Stamp)		
C. P.		PHYSICIANS' ORDER SHEET

Date/Time	ORDERS
5/5/XX 7 a.m.	Transfer to PCCU today.
	Implement Phase II rehab program in PCCU, keep HR limit at 100.
	Low cholesterol diet.
	Valium 5 mg. t.i.d.
	NTG 1/100 gr. p.r.n. at bedside
	J.D. M.D.

References

1. WENGER, N. K., *Coronary Care—Rehabilitation After Myocardial Infarction* (New York: American Heart Association, 1973), pp. 18-25.
2. REILLY, D. E., *Behavioral Objectives in Nursing: Evaluation of Learner Attainment* (New York: Appleton-Century-Crofts, 1975), p. 4.
3. *Ibid.*
4. MAGER, R. F., *Preparing Instructional Objectives,* 2nd ed. (Belmont, California: Fearon-Pitman Publishers, 1975).
5. McASHAM, H., *Writing Behavioral Objectives* (New York: Harper & Row, Publishers, Inc., 1970).

9

implementation of phase II cardiac rehabilitation

Behavioral Objectives

After completion of this chapter, the reader should be able to:

- name the usual members of the rehab team and briefly describe the role of each.
- discuss how physical location affects Phase II rehab implementation.
- outline a plan for collection of patient education supplies.
- begin a list of policies and procedures needed to implement a Phase II program.

Introduction

Concentrated individualized education, progressive activity, and continued support are nursing functions basic to Phase II cardiac rehab. Planning is, of course, the preparation for and selection of how to meet patient needs through such nursing functions. Implementation is bringing the plan to life and making it work. The thought processes of planning are continuous with the action processes of implementation. To make the conversion from thought to action requires a general structure and form within which an effective Phase II rehab program can be developed.

Program Design Considerations

Personnel Roles

One of the first questions to be answered about Phase II program design is who should be involved. The answer will depend upon program philosophy, resources available, and medical and administrative policies of the sponsoring institution.

The Patient and Family. Ideally, every cardiac rehab program philosophy contains the commitment that the patient is an equal partner in his health care. The patient and his significant others, then, are the first "personnel" considered essential in constructing an inpatient rehab program.

Active participation of patients in health care planning and provision is still novel. For the ideal to become actual requires education not only of the patient-participant, but also of the other program personnel. Health care professionals used to functioning in roles in which the patient was a passive recipient of care may have difficulty adjusting to giving their patients "equal time."

Nurse Coordinator. The professional who plans, coordinates, implements, and evaluates the rehab program as a whole is usually the nurse with cardiac rehab specialty training and experience. Nurse coordinator or director responsibilities include

1. Patient care—Seeing that each patient's rehab needs are identified, that a rehab plan is developed to meet those needs, and that the plan is well executed and evaluated.
2. Program management—Defining staff responsibilities, facilitating communication, scheduling patient assignments and working hours, and so on.
3. Professional guidance—Assuring that program procedures are based on the most current scientific information and that all health professionals are informed through appropriate continuing education.

In smaller institutions, the nurse coordinator may assume responsibility for direct patient care as well as for the above supervisory functions. In larger hospitals with a heavy volume of cardiac patients, active involvement of many staff nurses is needed. Ideally, all nurses working with postmyocardial infarction patients should have a functional knowledge of the principles and procedures of activity progression and patient education. Phase II cardiac rehabilitation could then be implemented by any nurse with the guidance of the nurse coordinator. This approach coincides with the philosophy of primary care nursing.

Physicians. The *physician director* of an inpatient cardiac rehab program has the responsibility of overseeing the medical care given to Phase II patients. His functions are similar to those of the CCU director and, in fact, frequently the same physician holds both positions.

The physician director position also involves educating primary care physicians in the purposes and rationale of therapeutic techniques used in cardiac rehab and serving as authoritative resource to other health   professionals.

The patient's attending physician, or *primary care physician*, is the person who must write orders for those components of cardiac rehab care that are considered medical therapy (for example, activity progression, medications, diet, and so on). To do so requires that he be informed about program availability, program services, and his/her role. The primary care physician knows the patient and his family, their problems, their strengths and weaknesses, and their resources. His/her input should be sought and active participation throughout the patient's rehabilitation encouraged.

Other Health Professionals. Involvement of other health professionals depends upon their availability and training. Figure 9-1 is a schematic representation of the various roles of health care personnel in Phase II cardiac rehabilitation.

Personnel Relationships

The combination of people in any or all of the rehab roles just described is generally called the rehab "team." The concept of team as used in the design of an inpatient cardiac rehab program should be specifically defined. Matheson, Selvester, and Rice effectively discuss the differences between team approaches. **The Interdisciplinary Team** is one in which decisions are made jointly by members, and each discipline accepts the peer status of the other.[P] Advantages of this approach are the accessibility and the integration of all patient care services. Problems involved in utilizing the interdisciplinary approach include coordinating the time and availability of as many as six to twelve busy health professionals.

The Multidisciplinary Team is one in which the members do not have well-integrated decisions, and professional status rather than equal participation continues to dominate.[2]

Though less ideal, this is the "team" that seems to occur most often, frequently by default. That is, an institution may philosophically subscribe to the interdisciplinary concept, but obstacles encountered in its organization and implementation erode the idealism. The compensatory result, the multidiscipline approach, can be implemented effectively if the team "coordinator" is equally knowledgeable in rehab care and personnel management.

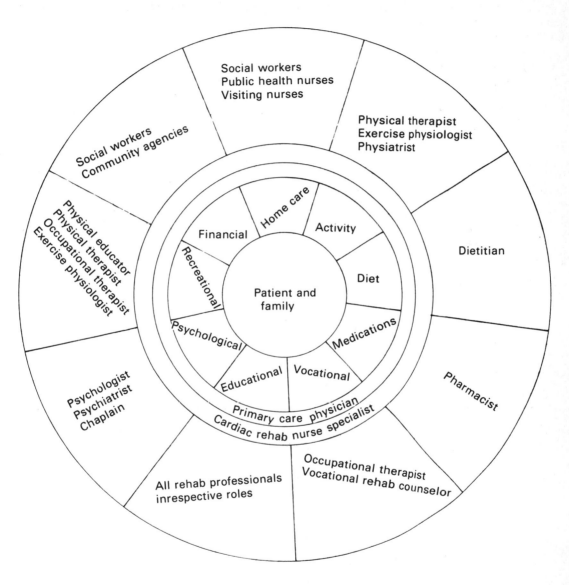

Figure 9-1. Roles of health professionals in Phase II cardiac rehabilitation.

Program Location

Roles and relationships just discussed are related to and sometimes dependent upon the location chosen for the Phase II rehab program. References to patient care and cardiac rehab activities throughout Unit II state or imply that the events discussed take place in the subspecialty environment of a progressive unit. This intermediate unit is the ideal setting for implementing an organized inpatient cardiac rehab program.

However, the goals of Phase II rehab can be accomplished without a shining new subspecialty unit. In hospitals where because of space, financial problems, or general medical philosophy patients are transferred from CCU directly to a medical floor, the same rehab plan can be effectively implemented with some added nursing effort. Nursing assessments may need to be more inclusive and/or frequent since the patient is in a less visible environment. The nurse specialist will have to assume responsibility for orienting and assisting the nurses on the floor staff who will be responsible for the patient's daily care. Functions need to be delineated. In this location, primary nursing would seem to be the nursing approach of choice to enhance cardiac rehab.

Program Equipment

The biggest equipment cost and consideration in organizing a Phase II program is that of continuous monitoring. Should patients be monitored 24 hours a day in Phase II as they were in Phase I? Or should they only be monitored during performance of new activities? Or can some objective guideline other than ECG monitoring be used to evaluate performance?

Since almost one-third of inhospital cardiac deaths occur after the patient's transfer from CCU,[3] the possibility that ECG surveillance continued into the postacute period of hospitalization may identify early rhythm abnormalities and prevent a number of cardiac arrests cannot be overlooked. Unfortunately, the occurrence or severity of ventricular arrhythmias in CCU does not indicate patients likely to experience rhythm abnormalities later in hospitalization.[4]

Conventional bedside monitors like those used in most CCUs are not applicable to progressive units since the short patient cables would not allow for monitoring during Phase II activities. The ECG telemetry systems, though generally more expensive than hard-wired bedside monitors, are the monitoring equipment of choice for intermediate CCUs (Chapter 14 offers a detailed description of telemetry use). Figure 9-2 shows samples of telemetry strips recorded during Phase II activities.

A "satellite" monitor has been used in some units where continuous telemetry is not available for all patients. The small portable monitor is taken to the area where the patient will be performing a prescribed activity. He is hooked up to the telemetry and monitored throughout the performance. Activity strips obviously provide performance assessment information and on occasion may provide identification of high-risk rhythm abnormalities.

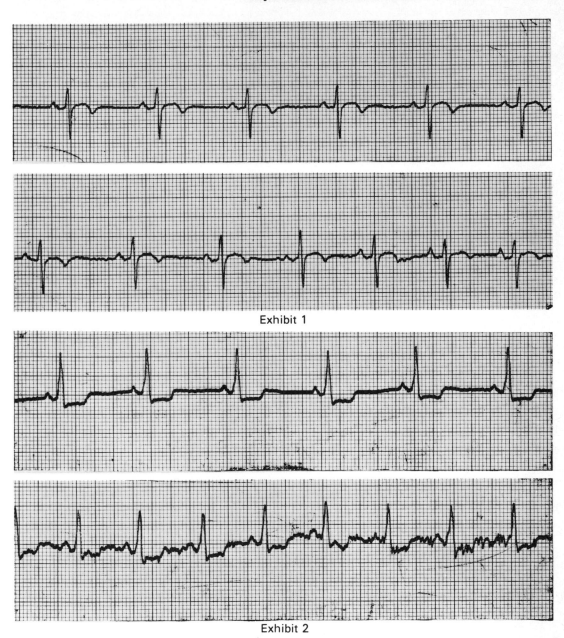

Exhibit 1

Exhibit 2

Figure 9-2.   Telemetry recordings during Phase II activity.

Program Materials

Because of the educational emphasis of Phase II nursing care, a variety of educational materials needs to be assembled. Chapter 8 reviewed useful types of teaching aids and sources.

During program organization, certain determinations relative to patient educational planning should be made.

Supply Budget. What funds are available for purchase and replenishment of patient educational materials? Will materials used be charged to patients or included in their hospital costs?

What sources of financial aid are available outside of the general budget to help defray supply costs (for example, hospital auxiliary or volunteer group projects)? What inhouse equipment, supplies, or talents already available could be converted to patient education use (for example, audiovisual equipment, medical art departments, librarians, and so on)?

What community agencies have materials or personnel available for patient education services free of charge (such as, American Lung Association speakers on smoking, an array of valuable material from American Heart Association, and the like)?

What health professionals already on the hospital staff can supply ideas and advice on inhouse "designer's original" patient educational material?

Material Approval. What person and/or committee needs to review and approve patient educational materials before they can be used for program teaching? Do master educational plans need to be written and reviewed prior to initiation of teaching?

Policies

As with any inhospital nursing service, policies must be developed to guide the nursing functions involved with Phase II cardiac rehab. The following areas of policy should be definitive: Which patients will be admitted to the Progressive Coronary Unit? Which patients will participate in the Phase II program? All? Only those by physician's order? Which program components require a physician's order for implementation?

Procedures

Some Phase II functions, such as activity progression, should be specified in a procedural format consistent with the format for nursing procedures throughout the hospital. Other functions, such as patient education, less readily lend themselves to sequential "how to" procedures, but depending upon nursing service policies, may require some type of written description. Care must be taken to assure that written teaching guidelines are organized sufficiently to standardize the teaching program while remaining flexible enough to individualize patient education.[5]

Documentation of Progress

Charting

Written documentation of rehab care is a nursing responsibility. Notations should include a record of procedures performed and/or activities carried out accompanied by a description of patient responses and adjustments made in the rehab plan (see Chapter 4 for discussion of charting format). Such charting is an ongoing report of progress. The sample case at the end of the chapter offers some examples.

Staff Communication

Discussion of roles and relationships in the preceding section mentioned the importance of communication among the professionals involved with the patient's rehab care. Verbal progress reports at scheduled team meetings may supplement, but should not replace, written information. Less formally, one-to-one updates between the nurse coordinator and another member of the rehab team should take place throughout the patient's Phase II involvement. Remembering that the patient is a member of the rehab team, evidence of progress or need for change should be shared with him as well.

(Patient ID Stamp)

C. P.	**CARDIAC REHAB PROGRESS NOTES**

Date/Time	PROGRESS NOTES
5/9/XX 3 p.m.	Phase II/Level 5:
	Preactivity assessment WNL
	S. Slightly fatigued, no SOB or chest pain. Accurately counted pre- and postactivity pulse.
	O. See activity flow sheet for responses. Walking in hall several times a day.
	A. Doing well with both activity and educational sessions. Wife in at lunch time for discussion with dietitian.
	P. Group session for patients/families on "Stress and Your Heart" by Dr. C. D. tomorrow evening. Patient and wife invited to attend.
	n. d., R.N.

(Patient ID Stamp)

C. P.	CARDIAC REHAB PROGRESS NOTES

5/11/XX 10:30 a.m.	Phase II/Level 7:
	No signs/symptoms prior to exercise.
	S. Very pleased with successful accomplishment of stair descent. Enjoyed group session last evening, requested stress booklets.
	O. No unusual responses (see activity sheet).
	A. Continues to progress well.
	P. Flexibility exercises to be performed mid-afternoon and evening. Will provide stress material this afternoon. Will check with Dr. J. D. re expected date of discharge.
	N.D., R.N.

CARDIAC ACTIVITY PROGRESSION FLOW SHEET

Name _____ C. P. _____ Phase ____ II ____ Physician _____ J. D. _____

Date / Level	HR	Preactivity Rhythm	BP	Rx Date / HR Limit — Activity Performed	Activity Response HR	Rhythm	BP	HR	Postactivity Rhythm	BP	Supervised By
Date: 5/9/XX Level: 5				Rx Date: 5/5/XX HR Limit: 100							
Time 3 p.m. Time Time	80	NSR	132/70	Stretching and flexibility exercises	90	NSR	144/70	84	NSR	130/70	h.l. R.N.
Date: Level:				Rx Date: ____ HR Limit: ____							
Time Time Time											
Date: 5/11/XX Level: 7				Rx Date: 5/11/XX HR Limit: 100							
Time 10 a.m. Time Time	74	NSR	132/70	Down 1 flight of stairs	84	NSR	140/78	76	NSR	136/68	n.l. R.N.
Date: Level:				Rx Date: ____ HR Limit: ____							
Time Time Time											
Date: Level:				Rx Date: ____ HR Limit: ____							
Time Time Time											
Date: Level:				Rx Date: ____ HR Limit: ____							
Time Time Time											

References

1. MATHESON, L. N., SELVESTER, R. H., and RICE, H. E., "The Interdisciplinary Team in Cardiac Rehabilitation," *Rehabilitation Literature*, December 1975, pp. 366-385.
2. *Ibid.*
3. GRACE, W. J., and YARVOTE, P. H., "Acute Myocardial Infarction: The Cause of the Illness Following Discharge From the Coronary Care Unit: A Description of the Intermediate Coronary Care Unit," *Chest*, Vol. 59, 1971, pp. 15-17.
4. BIGGER, J. T., et al., "Ventricular Arrhythmias in Ischemic Heart Disease: Mechanism, Prevalence, Significance, and Management," *Progress in Cardiovascular Diseases*, January-February 1977, pp. 255-300.
5. BOGGS, B., MALONE, D., and McCULLOCH, C., "A Coronary Teaching Program in a Community Hospital," *Nursing Clinics of North America*, Vol. 13, No. 3, (Philadelphia: W. B. Saunders Company, September 1978), pp. 457-472.

10

evaluation of phase II cardiac rehabilitation

Behavioral Objectives

After completion of this chapter, the reader should be able to:

- **give examples of the kinds of activity Phase II patients should be capable of by the time of discharge.**
- **state the purpose of predischarge exercise testing.**
- **suggest general guidelines for low-level exercise testing.**
- **discuss the use of behavioral objectives as a means of evaluating patient education.**
- **list at least five patient outcomes to be expected from an effective Phase II program.**
- **summarize Phase II discharge functions.**

Introduction

Effective Phase II cardiac rehabilitation programs are erasing the long-standing image of the patient who comes home as a cardiac cripple. The degree of each patient's discharge readiness reflects the effectiveness of Phase II. Measurement and documentation of such readiness is a nursing function. Information obtained through predischarge evaluation is helpful to the patient's rehab continuity as well as to the improvement of Phase II nursing care.

Evaluation of Patient Responses

As discussed in preceding chapters, planned activity progression enables the patient to slowly and safely resume performance of self-care and daily activities. The patient who is able to accomplish physical tasks equivalent to about three METs of energy expenditure at the time of discharge will return home able to care for himself and, therefore, be less dependent, less demanding, and less depressed. In addition to complete self-care and initiation of a daily walking program, types of activity generally allowable at a three MET level are shown in Table 10-1.

Table 10-1
Sample At Home Activities Requiring Approximately 3 METs

Casual Tasks	Casual Recreation
Driving a car	Badminton
Gardening	Bicycling
Light housework	Billards
Cooking	Bowling
Dusting	Canoeing
Ironing	Dancing
Making beds	Fishing
Mopping	Hiking
Sewing	Musical instruments
Sweeping	Table tennis
Washing clothes	
Light hand tools	
Typing	

METs relate to physical energy requirements only. Emotional factors accompanying any activity may raise the MET requirement. Adapted from "Cardiac Reconditioning and Work Evaluation Unit," *Exercise Equivalents*, (Denver, Colorado: Colorado Heart Association, p. 12; 1970), Fox, S. M., Naughton, J. P., and Gorman, P. A., "Physical Activity and Cardiovascular Health," *Modern Concepts of Cardiovascular Disease*, June 1972, p. 27; and American College of Sports Medicine, *Guidelines for Graded Exercise Testing and Exercise Prescription* (Philadelphia: Lea & Febiger, 1975), pp. 31, 37-40.

Predischarge Exercise Testing

Specific measurement of a patient's physical capability and corresponding cardiac responses is readily accomplished through predischarge exercise testing. Ordered and supervised by the physician, such testing identifies each patient's upper performance level and, thus, allows for specific discharge instructions regarding activities.

Test Performance. Exercise stress testing is a subscience of cardiology. Various types of tests and the techniques involved are described in detail in Chapter 17. Exercise testing as carried out prior to discharge is an application of the submaximal testing approach. That is, an arbitrary goal is set prior to the test toward which performance progresses. The predetermined goal is usually a moderate increase in heart rate response, such as 120 beats per minute[1] or a one-third increase over the resting heart rate.[2]

The test begins at a very low level of work and proceeds slowly. Treadmill protocols useful for predischarge testing are shown in Table 10-2.

Test Safety. The heart rate guidelines chosen as test endpoints were selected to enable collection of sufficient information to accomplish the test purpose, while at the same time maintaining patient safety. Several studies have demonstrated that predischarge testing when conducted by knowledgeable professionals using modest performance guidelines and responding to the earliest signs suggestive of cardiac difficulty is not a high-risk procedure.[3-6]

Table 10-2
Treadmill Protocols Useful for Predischarge Testing

Title		Test Levels	=	MET Levels		Level Duration
Lerman	I	1.2 mph 0 %	=	2	METs	
	II	1.2 mph 3 %	=	2.5	METs	Three minutes each
	III	1.2 mph 6 %	=	3	METs	
Naughton	I	2.0 mph 0 %	=	2	METs	
	II	2.0 mph 3.5 %	=	3	METs	Two minutes each
	III	2.0 mph 7 %	=	4	METs	

Adapted from Lerman, J., et al., "Low-level Dynamic Exercises for Earlier Cardiac Rehabilitation: Aerobic and Hemodynamic Responses," *Archives of Physical Medicine and Rehabilitation*, Volume 57, 1976, p. 355; and Naughton, J. P., "The Contribution of Regular Physical Activity to the Ambulatory Care of Cardiac Patients," *Postgraduate Medicine*, April 1975, p. 53.

Advantages of Predischarge Testing. The advantages of predischarge testing can be seen from two viewpoints, that of the patient and that of the nurse. For the nurse, test results provide specific guidelines within which individualized activity advice can be given and exercise performance implemented according to physician prescription.[7]

For the patient, test performance provides personal proof of capability. In some cases, the patient may be surprised at the extent of his performance. In others, the patient may be disappointed by his performance, but helped to realize the importance of his role in achieving rehab goals. Positive motivation may result in either case, enhancing rehab commitment and cooperation.

Predischarge Educational Assessment

Among many busy health professionals, there is a tendency to assume that because a patient has been taught, he has, in fact, learned. Such an assumption is erroneous. Giving of information, even the most up-to-date information using the most dramatic techniques available, in no way guarantees receipt of the information by the patient. Patient learning must be continually evaluated (see Chapter 8). Education should be arranged to provide plenty of time for teaching, evaluation, reinforcement, and reteaching if necessary prior to the time of discharge. The patient should have the opportunity to practice some of the skills he will be expected to perform by the time of discharge. For example, the patient should be observed accurately counting his pulse and modifying his activities so his heart rate does not exceed the set limitations.

Of course, the use of behavioral objectives enhances evaluation by predetermination of when and how patient learning will be measured. Just prior to discharge, a discussion period should be scheduled with patient and family to review learning achievements and identify remaining objectives. In instances where some objectives may not have been met, discussion may be encouraged, for example, if a patient has not yet resolved to stop smoking. In other cases, reteaching may need to be performed, for example, if the patient is not able to describe the relationship of his risk factors to his heart condition. Learning needs not met during Phase II can, thus, be mutually identified and subsequently communicated to the nurse specialist who will be seeing the patient in the outpatient cardiac rehabilitation program.

Evaluation may also help identify areas of program weakness. If a number of patients have failed to achieve a stop-smoking objective, in-depth evaluation should be made of the smoking educational program. Does the nurse educator need to upgrade her educational plan? Are more dynamic teaching aids needed? Or, would assistance from other health professionals improve results?

Expected Patient Outcomes

Gauging patient achievements through use of expected outcomes is a useful means of evaluation. Evaluation results can be used in conjunction with formal patient care audit procedures or simply as an achievement reference. Common patient outcomes useful in Phase II evaluation are listed in Table 10-3.

Table 10-3
Common Patient Outcomes of Phase II Cardiac Rehabilitation

Physiological Outcomes	Psychosocial Outcomes	Educational Outcomes
Upon discharge from the Phase II inpatient program, the cardiac patient should be able to:	Upon discharge from the Phase II inpatient program, the cardiac patient should be able to:	Upon discharge from the Phase II inpatient program, the cardiac patient should be able to:
Perform activities at an energy level equivalent to approximately three METs.	Describe feelings resulting from his change in health and express a realization that certain psychological changes are normal during recovery stages.	Describe coronary artery disease, describe myocardial infarction, and discuss their relationship.
Describe expected responses to allowable activities.	State a desire to continue participation in his own health care through an outpatient cardiac rehab program.	Name his personal risk factors and express a desire to pursue necessary habit changes.
		Discuss basic types of exercise and correctly relate differences to common activities of daily living.
		Accurately demonstrate pulse taking as a response assessment to increasing activities.
		Name each of his prescribed medications, and state their purpose, dosage, frequency and possible side effects.

Table 10-4
Predischarge Checklist

Verbal and/or written instructions pertinent to the following discharge items to be included in predischarge education:

Postdischarge Activities
_____ Driving
_____ Gardening
_____ Housework
_____ Recreation
_____ Sexual activity
_____ Social events
_____ Stair climbing
_____ Walking

Postdischarge Appointments
_____ Counseling services
_____ Outpatient cardiac rehab program
_____ Physician's office

Discharge Functions

Discharge is the culmination of assessment, planning, implementation, and evaluation of Phase II nursing care. In the process of cardiac rehabilitation, hospital discharge does not represent an end in itself, but rather a forward step toward an even greater health commitment—outpatient cardiac rehabilitation.

Evaluation of patient objectives and comparison to expected outcomes locates the patient's rehab position. As a reminder that all points of interest have been adequately covered, the nurse specialist may find a checklist of appropriate discharge items helpful (see Table 10-4).

Documentation of the patient's discharge status should recap the objectives met and list the needs remaining. The discharge summary format can follow the SOAP outline suggested for all nurse's notes. An example is shown in the sample case at the end of this chapter.

In hospitals where primary care nursing is practiced, rehab continuity is enhanced by having the same nurse follow the patient during both inpatient and outpatient rehab. Where different nurses are responsible for inpatient and outpatient cardiac rehab, continuity can be improved by thorough evaluation and documentation supplemented by a nursing transfer conference (see Chapter 12).

(Patient ID Stamp)

C. P.

**EXERCISE STRESS
TEST RESULTS**

Test Date   5/14/XX   **Time**   7:30 a.m.   **Purpose**   Predischarge evaluation

Testing Physician   J. D., M.D.   **Testing Nurse**   N. S., R.N.

Test Device/Protocol   Treadmill/mod. Naughton   **HR Guide**   120 submax.

Medications   Valium 5 mg. t.i.d.

Exercise Response Flow Chart

Work Stages	Cum. Time	Heart Rate	Blood Pressure	ST Segment	Other ECG Changes	Signs/ Symptoms
Baseline	—	75	120/76			
2 mph/0%	2	90	130/80			
2/3.5%	4	102	130/80	↓ .5 mm.		
2/7%	6	124	140/82	↓ .5 mm.	2 APCs	
Immediate		120		↓ .5 mm.		
2' recovery		96		↓ .5 mm.		
4' recovery		90		—		
6' recovery		84		—		

Reason(s) for terminating the test: Submaximal heart rate goal achieved

Recorded By: *n. s. R. n.*

(Patient ID Stamp)

C. P.

| **EXERCISE STRESS TEST**
| **PHYSICIAN'S INTERPRETATION**

5/14/XX   10 a.m.

TEST SUMMARY:

A low level exercise test was performed to determine a heart rate for postdischarge activities. Patient completed the 6 minute treadmill test without incident. Responses:

HR
B/P   } in line with work applied and stage of recovery

ECG: ST segment depression of 0.5 mm in line with healing; a few APC's at end of test unremarkable.

INTERPRETATION:

No abnormal exercise responses. Patient to be discharged tomorrow. Phase III outpatient rehab to begin next week. Heart rate limit for home and rehab activities at 120.

J.D., M.D.

(Patient ID Stamp)

C. P.	**CARDIAC REHAB PROGRESS NOTES**

Date/Time	PROGRESS NOTES
5/15/XX 10 a.m.	Discharge Summary:
	Objectives 1 through 5, 7, 8 achieved as noted on Rehab Plan. Diet related objectives (#6) need additional follow-up. Patient and wife have basic awareness but uncertain as to everyday implementation. Should be pursued further in Phase III.
	S. Patient was eager to carry out activities and learn all that was offered in Phase II. Stated he thinks he knows "how to handle myself at home." Attitude is optimistic.
	O. Phase II activity progress was without unusual incident. Can accurately count pulse to assess activity tolerance. No dysrhythmia or chest discomfort with increased activities. Predischarge exercise test tolerated well (see test results sheet). HR limit set at 120.
	A. Patient improved physically and emotionally as activities and education progressed. He has a good understanding of what has happened and what he must do to continue to improve after discharge.
	P. Has been scheduled for first outpatient visit of Phase III on Tuesday. Toured the exercise unit and met outpatient nurses yesterday in conjunction with exercise test. Has appointment with Dr. J. D. in 2 weeks.
	Will give verbal report on patient at tomorrow's transfer conference.

R.J. R.N.

References

1. ERICSSON, M., et al., "Arrhythmias and Symptoms During Treadmill Testing 3 Weeks After Myocardial Infarction in 100 Patient," *British Heart Journal,* Vol. 35, 1973, pp. 787-790.
2. SIVARAJAN, E., et al., "Low Level Treadmill Testing of 41 Patients With Acute Myocardial Infarction Prior to Discharge from the Hospital," *Heart and Lung,* November-December 1977, pp. 975-980.
3. ERICSSON, *op. cit.,* pp. 787-790.
4. SIVARAJAN, *op. cit.,* pp. 975-980.
5. LERMAN, J., et al., "Low-level Dynamic Exercises for Earlier Cardiac Rehabilitation: Aerobic and Hemodynamic Responses," *Archives of Physical Medicine and Rehabilitation,* Vol. 57, p. 355.
6. JOHNSTON, B. L., et al., "Sexual Activity in Exercising Patients After Myocardial Infarction and Revascularization," *Heart and Lung,* November-December 1978, p. 1029-1031.
7. *Ibid.*

unit III

phase III
cardiac
rehabilitation

11

background and basics of phase III cardiac rehabilitation

Behavioral Objectives

After completion of this chapter, the reader should be able to:

■ state the purpose of a Phase III cardiac rehab program.

■ discuss the health care advantages of continuing professional contact into the immediate postdischarge period.

■ list six nursing capabilities specifically applied in Phase III care.

■ explain the cause of posthospital depression commonly experienced by postmyocardial infarction patients.

■ describe three feelings family members frequently experience following patient discharge.

Introduction

Hospital discharge is a joyful event. But, for most postmyocardial infarction patients, the happiness of returning home quickly fades as the realities of life make themselves known once again. The patient did not live in protective isolation before being hospitalized, and he cannot be expected to remain in a restrictive cocoon after discharge.

Returning home can be thought of as re-entry into the world of everyday living, a world of people—spouse, family, boss, coworkers, friends, neighbors; places—home, work, community; events—births/deaths, holidays, income tax, growing older, winning/losing; and emotions—love/hate, frustration/satisfaction. Successful re-entry is a two-step procedure. The first step is advance preparation through extensive teaching and discharge planning as done in Phase II. The second step is continuing support and professional assistance through each area of re-entry. This kind of ongoing contact is provided in a Phase III program.

Purpose

One of the goals expressed in the cardiac rehabilitation definition is the achievement and maintenance of optimal psychosocial health. The purpose of an organized Phase III cardiac rehab program is to emphasize striving toward that goal. An optimal psychosocial level is difficult to specifically define because what is best psychologically and socially is relative to each patient. Optimal in a psychosocial sense might be defined as having a functional and meaningful daily life. This concept includes acceptance of self and satisfactory relationships with family, peers, and society at large.

Helping the patient to safely resume his normal life-style or to find more acceptable substitutes is a major step toward the psychosocial goal. Too often in the past, patients were "discharged in good health" to make their own sick-to-well transition. Visits to their doctor's office helped with physical problems that arose, but provided little, if any, psychosocial assistance.

A Phase III cardiac rehab program takes place during the immediate post-discharge period, but is continuous with the Phase II inpatient program proximally and the Phase IV outpatient program distally. Usually conducted from the outpatient cardiac rehab unit, the Phase III setting is ideally introduced to the patient prior to discharge. As part of discharge preparation, the patient could be taken to the outpatient unit to be introduced to the staff and given a tour of the facilities. To most patients, this "preview of coming attractions" is encouraging, promoting expectations of improvement.

Equally important in easing discharge anxieties is the patient's awareness that a knowledgeable health professional will be available to answer his questions and provide gentle reminders if he forgets any of the discharge instructions. It is comforting to know where and whom to call just in case a problem arises.

Nursing Requisites

The nurse, more than any other health professional, is in a position to effectively assist the patient through his posthospital transition. She has seen him through his acute illness and early recovery, knows his health problems and personal concerns, and is prepared to mobilize resources appropriate to the patient's needs.

Awareness of common psychosocial concerns, methods of handling them successfully, and alternatives available comprise the specialized knowledge base needed for Phase III nursing. Technical capability for handling various ambulatory monitoring equipment is also necessary. Table 11-1 gives an overview of Phase III nursing requirements. Subsequent chapters discuss each function in detail.

Table 11-1
Specialized Nursing Requirements for Phase III Cardiac Rehabilitation

Cognitive	Psychomotor

Basic awareness of psychological effects of serious illness
    On patient
    On significant others
	Operation of ambulatory monitoring equipment
	    Telemetry
	    Holter systems

Recognition of social implications of cardiac disease
    Sexual function
    Work performance
    Community reaction	

Promotion of behavioral changes
    Medication compliance
    Smoking withdrawal
    Dietary adjustments
    Appropriate exercise	

The Psychosocial Basis of Phase III

The psychological effects of serious illness and the sociological influences on recovery are both complex issues within complex sciences. In-depth descriptions of the psychology and sociology of cardiac patients are beyond the scope of this text. However, since a basic understanding of what is going on *inside* the postmyocardial infarction patient (psychology) and what is going on in the *outside* world, but having a direct effect upon him (sociology), is essential to effective Phase III nursing, the following review is offered.

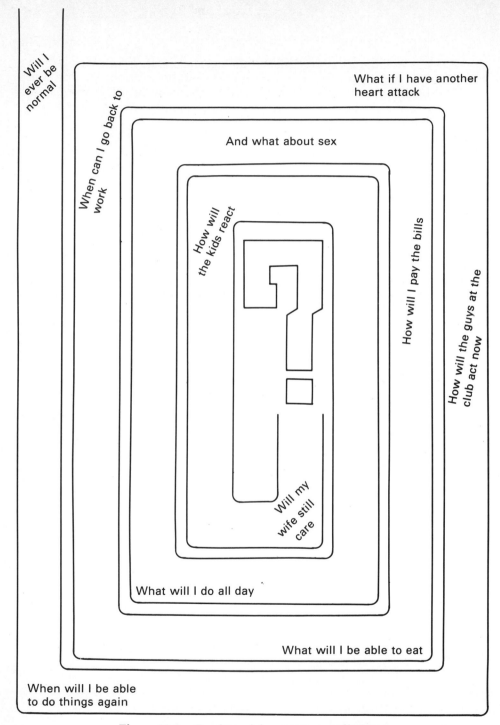

Figure 11-1. Psychosocial concerns postdischarge.

The Patient's Experience

The search for "self" is a constant universal struggle. Progress gained in a person's lifetime may be quickly diminished by disease with its standard accompaniments of life-threats and ego-insults. The task of rebuilding ego strength and ultimately self-concept needs to be diligently pursued as the patient progresses toward optimal recovery. If the patient is unable to fulfill his normal roles, those consistent with his self-concept, he will feel frustrated and inadequate. Defensive behavior will result and rehabilitation will be hindered.

It is common for the cardiac patient to feel well prior to discharge from the hospital and immediately upon returning home find himself overcome with feelings of weakness, depression, and anxiety. This change can be exaggerated by the interpretation of these signs as a relapse or deterioration of his condition. Being forewarned of this likely occurrence with supplemental advice to rest adequately, exercise appropriately, and take psychotropic drugs if prescribed will contribute to a less traumatic transition for patient and family.

Posthospital feelings of depression are understandable considering that at this time more than any other the patient and family are directly faced with the problems of restructuring their lives. Implications of the cardiac event on their lives may seem monumental. This is the time when the patient realizes he has lost his health, confidence, and independence. He is further confused by being asked to change old patterns of living which he may have found very satisfying: eating, drinking, smoking, and his sedentary hobby of watching television (see Figure 11-1).

Wishnie and associates[1] described high percentages of patients experiencing distress characterized by weakness, frustration, disturbed sleep, persistent insomnia, fear of having another myocardial infarction, corrosive conflict in families over implications of the illness, and other problems. Many of these patients needed tranquilizers or antidepressants, but the majority would not request medication from their physician either from fear of "getting hooked" or because they equated emotions with weakness or loss of virility.

Community and occupational reactions to heart disease may be added sources of distress to the patient. The understanding and acceptance of both employer and coworkers may mean the difference between the patient contemplating early return to work or struggling with long hours of fear and uncertainty as to whether he will be required to do more than he feels capable of performing.

Work is more than earning a living. Work frequently carves patterns of interpersonal associations and activities in the life of the patient. The patient's family may be organized around his work. It is little wonder that work is a major concern for most patients.

The Family's Experience

As a result of the patient's heart attack, the family has experienced significant loss—loss of security. Financial instability may add to the sense of loss. Having certain needs consistently filled establishes a routine life-style, the services of which may have been totally supplied by the patient. The family members may now find themselves in the supportive role where previously they were the ones supported by the patient. Anger and resentment may result.

Family members may be experiencing feelings of guilt regarding the cause of the myocardial infarction. Feelings of having been too demanding, of not being supportive enough, or of contributing to recent arguments and chronic tensions in the family are not infrequent.

Sociological problems are interwoven with the patient's and family's process of coping with life during this period. Within the family itself there may be feelings of resentment by some family members because the patient is no longer able to totally fill his usual role. Simultaneously, the patient may resent his wife's being overprotective. Frustration and humiliation are common in the patient who feels he is too closely supervised in normal everyday activities. On the other hand, if the wife limits her concern, she is likely to be resented as being unsympathetic.

These postdischarge reactions and concerns are complicated issues interweaving emotions, personalities, and needs of the patient and all those whose lives touch his. There are no easy answers in dealing with the real problems now facing the patient. How the patient and family are able to cope with their situation will mirror to a large extent how they handled other stressful situations in their lives. They may confront the situation, deny it, be drawn closer together, or withdraw from each other and the real world.

It is suggested that the best way to help the patient and family cope is through education and activity.[2-3] An organized Phase III program can provide the education needed and the activity appropriate during this highly vulnerable time.

References

1. WISHNIE, H. A., HACKETT, T. P., and CASSEM, N. H., "Psychological Hazards of Convalescence Following MI," *JAMA*, Vol. 215, No. 8, 22 February 1971, pp. 1292-1296.
2. HASKELL, W., "Physical Activity After Myocardial Infarction," *American Journal of Cardiology*, 20 May 1974, pp. 776-782.
3. HACKETT, T. P. and CASSEM, N. H., "The Psychologic Reaction of Patients in the Pre and Post Hospital Phases of Myocardial Infarction," *Postgraduate Medicine*, Vol. 57, No. 5, April 1975, pp. 43-46.

12

assessments for phase III cardiac rehabilitation

Behavioral Objectives

After completion of this chapter, the reader should be able to:

- discuss the purposes of record review and a transfer conference prior to Phase III initiation.
- outline a useful approach for taking an outpatient nursing history.
- give at least five examples of symptoms likely to be identified by history having direct rehab implications.
- describe the type of job best evaluated by each of the following vocational assessment methods: energy expenditure matching, job simulation, on-the-job monitoring.
- list at least ten factors, other than the type of work itself, that directly influence the amount of energy required to perform a job.

Introduction

As the first half of a total outpatient program, Phase III ideally begins prior to discharge. That is, as part of discharge planning, the physician writes the order for the patient to begin the Phase III cardiac rehab program immediately after discharge. The Phase II nurse specialist then arranges a predischarge visit to the outpatient department, and his first outpatient appointment is made for three to five days after discharge. The transfer from inpatient to outpatient is thus accomplished smoothly and easily.

In some cases, however, the patient may have been hospitalized in another facility, either across town or out of state. He may return home after discharge without the advantages of having participated in a well-structured inpatient program. To begin this patient in the Phase III outpatient program requires a direct admission order from his physician.

In either situation, Phase III health care begins with a thorough nursing assessment.

Review of Hospital Records

Prior to the patient's first outpatient visit, a copy of the records from his recent hospitalization is obtained and closely reviewed by the nurse. Particular attention is paid to the following record areas.

Past Medical History

The past medical history may give clues to the current problem, educational needs, and special considerations. Usually included are past illnesses and hospitalizations; diagnoses and treatment; allergies, including food, drug, and contact; injuries, along with dates, special treatment and disability, if any; surgical procedures; past infectious diseases and childhood diseases.

A history of diabetes, hypertension, or hyperlipoproteinemia alerts the nurse to assess the patient's level of knowledge about these conditions, the relationship between the disease and the cardiovascular system, and the patient's compliance to his prescribed treatment plan.

Family History

Family history includes immediate blood relatives—mother, father, siblings, and children. Information should be available as to age, sex, and health status of living family members. Age and cause of death should be noted for deceased family members.

A family history of coronary artery disease, myocardial infarction, diabetes, hypertension, or hyperlipoproteinemia is especially significant to the cardiac patient. If any of these conditions are present, assessment should be planned to determine the patient's understanding of these conditions as risk factors to coronary artery disease.

Predischarge Exercise Test Results

As discussed in Chapter 10, the purpose of conducting a low-level exercise test prior to discharge is to provide an objective guideline for the extent of activity that can be safely performed upon discharge. The response limit identified by the test will be used to guide exercises performed during Phase III, to assess vocational potential, and to advise daily activities.

Discharge Summaries

Medical. What medical regimens was the patient placed on that may require nursing follow-up?

For example, if the patient went home with 0.25 mg. of digoxin prescribed daily, nursing follow-up in Phase III should include assessment of the patient's understanding of the medicine's purpose, correct methods of taking it, and side effects. If the patient did not receive any medication instruction prior to discharge, a basic teaching session on his medicines would be a Phase III priority.

As another example, if the patient was discharged on a prudent diet, does he know what that means? Has his wife been instructed in shopping and cooking tips? A teaching session may need to be scheduled with the dietitian.

Nursing. What rehab objectives were not met prior to discharge and why? Could the objectives be achieved in Phase III? Should they be modified?

For example, if the patient while still in CCU was advised by his physician to stop smoking, but promptly resumed smoking when transferred to the step-down unit (in spite of formidable instruction and an array of pamphlets on the dangers of smoking provided by the nurse specialist), should nursing efforts continue toward achieving the no-smoking objective? Yes! Phase III may be able to muster added support for the patient through peer groups or may simply reinforce information at a time when the patient is more receptive.

The Transfer Conference

In most facilities where all four phases of rehab care are offered, inpatient and outpatient programs are separate nursing functions. To facilitate smooth patient transfer and continuity of nursing care, a transfer conference is held between inpatient and outpatient nurses.

As with review of the patient's records, the nurses' meeting should take place before the patient's first outpatient visit. The meeting serves a two-way purpose. For the inpatient nurse, the transfer conference allows for presentation of a discharge report and a summary of the patient's remaining health care needs. Although this information will have been documented on the patient's chart, the nurse-to-nurse session provides for additional expression of patient care ideas or suggestions and contributes to mutual problem solving.

For the outpatient nurse, the transfer conference provides an opportunity to obtain clarification of any unclear record information or to ask specific questions about the patient's nursing care. Advice is frequently requested from the inpatient nurse on how to proceed in specific problem areas. Successful transfer is a joint nursing effort.

The Outpatient Nursing History

It is as important to understand the nature of the person who has a disease as it is to understand the nature of the disease the person has. Review of the patient's chart complemented by a transfer conference may facilitate the latter, whereas a comprehensive nurse-patient interview is the first step toward the former awareness.

A well-conducted interview will aid the development of rapport between nurse and patient, and at the same time, demonstrate the nurse's interest, understanding, and desire to foster a working relationship. The establishment of open communications will be important to all subsequent interactions.

Most of the subjective information desired in the initial assessment can be obtained via effective patient interview; communication skills and observation are the primary techniques required for interviewing. Appropriate use of these skills will enable the nurse to identify the physical, psychosocial, and educational needs of the patient.

Factors that may influence health care planning may also be uncovered. These may include the patient's basic strengths and weaknesses, the significant others in the patient's life who may be supportive in the treatment plan, and socioeconomic factors.

The interviewing segment of assessment is directed toward collection of subjective information that plays a fundamental part in planning future health care. The interview is best performed as part of the initial outpatient visit. This provides an opportunity to inform the patient of his role in health care planning and to answer any questions he may have. The patient not only has a right to know and understand his treatment plan, but the enlightened patient will feel less anxious and more cooperative.

The goals of the nurse-patient interview, then, are to open communication, to establish a working relationship, to provide an opportunity for observation and data collection, and to enable the patient to have his questions answered. Achievement of these goals can be anticipated only if the interview itself is well planned. Advance consideration should be given to appropriate interviewing techniques and factors which will enhance interviewing productivity (detailed description can be found in Unit II, Chapter 7).

Interview Design

Introduction. The greeting of the patient and others accompanying him is important in setting the tone for the interview to follow. The introduction should include the following:

- A personal introduction and statement of your role: "Good morning Mr. and Mrs. Smith; I am Jane Doe, a staff nurse here in the outpatient department, and I will be seeing you during your visits."
- An indication of the purpose of the interview and the time alloted: "I would like to spend the next 30 minutes or so talking with you and asking for some health information that will help us determine a treatment plan especially for you. I will also try to answer any questions you may have."

The brief introduction is usually followed by a review of the patient's vital statistics as gathered from the medical records, but possibly requiring expansion or correction. This discussion of nonthreatening information will allow the patient the time he may need to relax in this strange situation.

Body. The body is the part of the interview in which the subjective assessment is accomplished. The nurse should be well organized, preferably using a specific format of topics to be investigated. Information should be accurately recorded when given and clarifying questions asked. Organization, good communication skills, alertness to stated and implied data, and awareness of patient body language comprise the talents used by the effective interviewer. In addition to collecting information during this segment of the interview, the nurse should communicate her interest and offer assistance where indicated. The body of the interview should be the beginning of a working relationship between the nurse and the patient.

Conclusion. If the introduction stated the expected length of the interview and the fact that questions would be answered, the groundwork has been laid for an effective conclusion. The patient should be asked if questions have been answered to his satisfaction. He should understand that the interview has been one step in a total assessment leading to a program of education and exercise designed specifically for his needs, tolerances, and personality.

Optimism should be the prevailing feeling at the conclusion of the interview. More than any other part of the interview, the conclusion will influence the patient's attitude toward the nurse and the concept of rehabilitation that may have far-reaching efforts on subsequent interactions.

Suggested Format

Vital Statistics. Includes name (and nickname if appropriate), address, age, sex, race, marital status, educational level, occupation, work and home phone numbers, and significant others.

Many patients are more comfortable being addressed by their given name or nickname rather than the formal "Mr. Smith" in a situation such as the outpatient rehab program where a long-term working relationship will develop. A large percentage of nurses also find that being on a friendly first name basis helps foster the feeling of mutual respect and teamwork desirable in every rehabilitation plan.

Chief Complaint and Cardiac History. The patient recently discharged may or may not be experiencing symptoms at the time of the interview. All present symptoms and/or those related to the cardiac event should be identified. Indicate to the patient that information concerning his cardiac experience is important, but allow him to describe it in his own words, for example, "Can you tell me about your problem, starting with the first time you noticed any symptoms?"

The patient's dissertation should then be guided in such a way that it includes the time and manner of symptom onset, the characteristics of the symptoms, the precipitating factors if any, the action taken, and sequelae. This same process should be followed for each symptom or complaint the patient describes.

General State of Health. By questioning the patient about his general health, it is frequently possible to elicit his feelings about his health and prognosis. The patient's affect concerning his health may be a strong influence on how he will respond to his rehab plan.

Review of Systems. In questioning the patient regarding the various body systems, the nurse is searching for symptoms that may be relevant to the present illness, other problems the patient may be experiencing but has not mentioned since they seem unrelated to his heart, symptoms that may concern his future health or influence his ability to perform exercise, and topics about which the patient may need health education.

A systematic approach is recommended beginning with the statement of general health and progressing through each body system from the head toward the feet.

Table 12-1 presents a synopsis of subjective information that may be solicited during the nursing history. Symptoms identified are pertinent to cardiac rehab in that they highlight problems that could affect exercise performance or that require patient education.

Table 12-1
Sample of Rehab-Related Health Information Solicited Via
Nursing History Review of Systems

Skin	Ulcers and sores may indicate arterial insufficiency or diabetes mellitus. Sweating can occur in instances of a rapid fall in blood glucose. Additional symptoms of hypoglycemia may include weakness, tachycardia, headache, hunger, and neurological signs such as mental confusion and/or irritability. Dryness or coarseness of the skin may indicate hypothyroidism.
Head	The characteristic hypertension headache is throbbing in nature, usually in the occipital region. Headaches brought on by stress or increased activity may also indicate hypertension.
Eyes	Symptoms of visual impairment may be indicative of diabetes mellitus or retinal arteriosclerosis.
Ears	Problems with the acoustic nerve or labyrinth may cause symptoms of vertigo or tinnitus. This may preclude use of the treadmill as a mode of exercise testing or training due to the danger of loss of balance and falling.
Nose	Nasal discharge may indicate rhinitis, sinusitis, or allergies. Patients with this symptom may be taking medications which could affect their physiologic responses to exercise.
Respiratory	Dyspnea, orthopnea, or cough may be symptoms of congestive heart failure, a contraindication to exercise. COPD decreases the amount of oxygen available, and patients with any type of obstructive pulmonary disease have a decreased exercise tolerance. A smoking history should be taken and the patient's level of knowledge regarding the physiological effect of smoking determined if he has this habit. What is his attitude about ceasing this habit?

Table 12-1
Sample of Rehab-Related Health Information Solicited Via
Nursing History Review of Systems

Cardiovascular	Any type of chest discomfort should be thoroughly investigated. People perceive pain differently; thus, a variety of terminology in soliciting information is useful. If the nurse calls symptoms "chest discomfort" rather than "pain," the patient may describe symptoms which are uncomfortable or disturbing but not actually painful as he perceives pain. Other useful terms include burning, indigestion, pressure, numbness, tingling, and aching. The presence of referred pain is also important—pain in the arm, neck, jaw, back, and between the shoulder blades. Has there been a change in the pain pattern of the angina patient? A change for the worse may be heralding a myocardial infarction. A history of rheumatic fever and/or heart murmur would alert the examiner to possible heart or valve disease. Palpitations, rhythm disturbances, or history of dysrhythmias is important. Are these associated with stimulants such as coffee, cola, exercise, or excitement? Does the patient experience associated symptoms such as vertigo, loss of consciousness, or chest discomfort with these symptoms? Does he have a history of hyperthyroidism?
Gastrointestinal	Weight gain or loss and ideal body weight may be discussed. Is the patient following a prescribed diet, does he understand the diet, and can he manage it? What is his attitude toward following the diet and his level of understanding of its management and influence on his cardiovascular condition? If the patient is on thiazide diuretics, what is his level of understanding regarding potassium replacement and salt restriction? If the patient is on Coumadin, does he realize the importance of avoiding foods high in vitamin K?
Metabolic	Does the diabetic patient have a good understanding of his disease and its management? Does he realize that exercise may call for some compensation in his diabetes management, and is he aware of his role in helping to assess his symptoms?
Genitourinary	Nocturia may be a symptom of congestive heart failure, uncontrolled diabetes mellitus, or taking diuretics incorrectly. The presence of any urinary problem such as polyuria, highly concentrated urine or oliguria may be associated with vascular problems and should be investigated. Returning to sexual activity is a concern for many patients. It is appropriate to question the patient on information he has received in this regard and supplement this information when necessary. A variety of medications, particularly antihypertensive drugs, have a side effect of causing impotence, and the patient should be questioned in such a way that this problem is identified when present.

Psychosocial History. The psychosocial history deals with the patient's lifestyle and self-concept. It attempts to identify his habits, beliefs, attitudes, significant others, and other things meaningful to the patient. Plans for behavioral changes in the patient's health interest will only be fruitful if implemented within the framework of his psychosocial situation.

Information should be obtained relevant to the following topics: usual sleep patterns, hobbies, exercise, sports, medications (both prescribed and over-the-counter drugs) taken regularly, alcohol use, tobacco use, recent losses, financial problems, relationships with family, relationship with others, religion, and usual reactions to a difficult situation. Much of this information may have already been provided during preceding parts of the interview. In addition to determining the patient's psychosocial status, the nurse needs to assess the patient's level of knowledge about the relationship of his habits and/or attitudes to coronary artery disease. Many educational needs may be uncovered during this portion of the interview.

Marital status is an obvious part of the psychosocial history. Marital status not only refers to being married, but to the status of that marriage. It is important to determine how supportive the spouse and other family members will be in helping the patient live his treatment plan. The spouse (or other significant person) should be included in the planning and educational sessions and given a good working knowledge of how to assist the patient.

The patient's and spouse's level of knowledge regarding sexual activity after myocardial infarction needs to be carefully investigated with special attention to discovering any misconceptions they harbor. An open-ended question such as, "what have you heard about returning to sexual activity after having had a heart attack?" is useful in ascertaining their awareness.

People are very sensitive about their knowledge of sex, seldom appreciating an inference that they are not knowledgeable enough or, worse still, that what they do believe is not correct. Diplomacy is essential for helping the patient to feel at ease. For example, if the patient indicates that he believes it is not customary for cardiac patients to be permitted to return to sexual activity, his information may be corrected by an explanation beginning with "many people believe that. Until recently, that was the instruction doctors were giving their patients. Since that time, studies have been done . . .", continuing with correct information.

Watts suggests that sexual assessment include the following information: sexual activity prior to the illness, general health of the patient and spouse, extent of recovery from the myocardial infarction, psychosocial needs of the spouse, and functioning of the marital unit.[1] Assessment of sexual knowledge, attitudes, and abilities as suggested, may best be approached in a forthright manner with progression from general to more explicit areas of sexual conduct. Information obtained will be helpful in establishing goals, planning methods of counseling, and identifying problems.

The quality of the marriage should also be determined. Sexual problems present prior to the cardiac event will probably still be present after the event and attempts to mend such a relationship between parties who do not truly desire it are likely to cause more stress for the patient and his spouse. The need for professional marriage counseling may be identified.

Occupational considerations are very important for the patient who is still in or anticipates returning to the labor force. What is the present employment status of the patient and what are his expectations for the future? There are many factors which could influence the patient's ability to perform his previous job. Patients who are currently employed or who are anticipating return to a previous position should be questioned about the components of that job (see Vocational Assessments).

Documentation. Information obtained through interviewing should be carefully documented and entered as a permanent record in the patient's outpatient chart. The written nursing history should conclude with a list of identified health problems that requires nursing intervention. Table 12-2 outlines a suggested method of documentation using the history format, oriented to a cardiac outpatient, discussed here.

Vocational Assessments

"When can I go back to work?" In the not too distant past, answers to this question depended on the subjective judgment of the physician. Most often, in the interest of patient safety, physicians were overconservative in selecting return-to-work dates.

In 1968, Kellerman reported that the majority of cardiac patients returned to work by five months postevent.[2] In 1973, Wenger reported results of a survey of U. S. physicians that indicated that over 85 percent of patients under age 65 returned to work within two to four months after uncomplicated myocardial infarctions.[3] The trend toward early return to work has been aided by the increasing availability of methods to objectively measure work energy expenditure. Patients can be told with more certainty when they are ready to undertake various work tasks.

Chronologically, the work question usually occurs in the early postdischarge period. Although addressed in generalities during Phase II, psychosocial concerns related to work often hit home soon after the patient's return. The nurse specialist in Phase III is a vital part of the work analysis team and is frequently involved with conducting job assessments.

Three types of job assessment are commonly used in conjunction with cardiac rehab programs.

Energy Expenditure Matching

Exercise testing measures work capacity. As discussed in Unit II, submaximal testing as performed before discharge stops at a predetermined heart rate level. The number of METs corresponding to the desired heart rate would be the patient's work capacity. Comparing the MET level achieved on the test to available metabolic cost tables, constructed from research of the oxygen cost of various occupational and recreational activities, a relationship between current capability and usual job requirement can be made.

For example, during his predischarge test, a patient achieves a heart rate of 125 beats per minute without difficulty. The treadmill work he performed was

Table 12-2
Nursing History Format

Vital Statistics

Name (and nickname)			Interview date
Age	Sex	Race	Marital status
Address			Home phone
Education			Religion
Significant others			
Referring physician			Phone
Place of employment			
Occupation			Work phone

Chief Complaint and/or Cardiac History

Symptoms (chest discomfort, leg cramps while walking, edema, difficulty breathing)
        Time and manner of symptom onset
        Characteristics of the symptom
        Precipitating factors, if any
        Action taken
        Sequelae

General State of Health

Fatigue, feeling of well-being, opinion about health

Review of Systems

Skin	-ulcers, sores, dryness, coarseness, diaphoresis
Head	-headaches
Eyes	-pain, visual impairment
Nose	-discharge, epistaxis
Respiratory	-dyspnea, orthopnea, COPD, smoking
Cardiovascular	-chest pain or discomfort; burning; indigestion; pressure; numbness; tingling; aching; pain in neck, jaw, back, and between the shoulder blades
Angina	-precipitating factors; characteristics; frequency; comparison of frequency to two weeks ago, two months ago, one year ago; effect of nitroglycerin, if used, and method of use
Gastrointestinal	-weight loss or gain, diet
Metabolic	-diabetic awareness
Genitourinary	-nocturia, polyuria, highly concentrated urine, oliguria

---

Past Medical History

Past illnesses, hospitalizations, diagnoses, and treatment
Allergies - drug, food, and contact; diabetes; hypertension;
hyperlipoprotenemia; obesity

Table 12-2
Nursing History Format

Medications

Prescribed and over-the-counter

Family History

	Age if living	Disease condition	Age at disease onset	Age at death	Cause of death
Mother					
Father					
Brothers					
Sisters					
Children					

Psychosocial

Usual sleep/relaxation patterns
Activities - hobbies, exercise sports
Alcohol
Tobacco
Recent losses
Financial problems
Relationship with family and others
Usual reaction or way of dealing with difficult situations
Occupation - present work status and future plans, components of job in rela-
        tion to stress, isometrics and environmental influences
Sexual patterns

Special Considerations

Impairments/influencing factors to education or exercise, attitude, learning ability, and so on.

Nursing Summary

Patient problems identified:
   1. (Example: stated that his "heart has a hole in it from the attack",
      and he "must rest until it grows over".)
   2. (Example: is still 20 lbs. overweight in spite of physician's
      instructions to lose weight)

Table 12-3
Work Circumstances Influencing Job Energy Requirements

Place	Performance	Psychological Stress
Access	Usual work pattern	Fear of loss of job if unable to "keep up"
Travel distance	Steady high level	Fear of cardiac emergency occurring on
Parking	Frequent high level	the job:
Public transportation	Occasional high level	Life threat
Heat	Steady low level	Job threat
Humidity	Usual work hours	Safety threat to others
Wind	Frequency of overtime	Fear of financial/seniority loss if change
Altitude	Isometric involvement	of job requested
Dust, smoke, or other airborne irritants	Pushing How	Fear of loss of group status if unable to
	Pulling Heavy?	do "equal share"
	Lifting	Fear of loss of family love and
	Carrying	community respect if any less a
	Degree of skill	"breadwinner"
	Personnel	
	Supervisor's attitude	
	Coworkers' acceptance	
	Responsibility for safety of others	
Pace		
Usual work speed		
Number and timing of rest intervals		
Production competition		
Deadlines/quotas		
Amount of travel		

equivalent to five METs. The patient is a self employed TV repairman. From the "Approximate Metabolic Cost of Activities,"[4] his type of job has been assigned to the two-to-three MET category. Matching the patient's test results to the job information, the objective conclusion is that, at least in terms of physical performance of the job, the patient will soon be able to return to work.

The biggest disadvantage of energy expenditure matching as just described may already be obvious. Translating test results to work performance does not take into account the influence of other physical and psychological factors on the energy that is needed. In drawing an assessment conclusion then, the work capacity measurement must be subjectively tempered by awareness of job circumstances. Much of this information is routinely obtained as part of the nursing history. Amplification of selected portions of the history may be necessary to complete the job assessment. Table 12-3 lists additional work influences to be evaluated.

Patients holding jobs with heavy physical requirements, such as laborers or construction workers where eight to nine METs of work is frequently required, will need to await a higher level of testing, such as is done to initiate Phase IV rehab, before their work assessment can be completed.

Job Simulation Performance

Since not all jobs have been classified into metabolic categories and since not all people perform the same job the same way, a more precise measurement of job energy expenditure, at least in terms of cardiovascular responses, may be obtained by actually having the patient perform his job or a very similar activity in the testing lab where his responses can be directly observed. Work evaluation units staffed with specially trained personnel to evaluate the patient's physical and psychological performance have been used for this purpose.[5] Consider again the TV repairman. If a faulty television set is brought into the lab and the patient is asked to actually fix it while being monitored, it may be discovered that the only time his heart rate exceeds 100 beats per minute is when he lifts the set. During this brief isometric action, his heart rate shoots to 135 and an occasional ventricular ectopic is seen on the monitor.

Results of this type of job assessment may be specific modification of those work tasks identified as threatening to the patient. In this case, is there an assistant who could do the occasional lifting that is necessary or could the sets be placed on a mobile cart to facilitate moving from place to place?

Another advantage of the job simulation approach is that it can look specifically at jobs requiring upper extremity involvement. Since most exercise testing is done using leg work, no evidence of upper extremity capability is derived. Assembly line machinists lifting and moving heavy equipment parts, for example, should have their job assessment with improvised upper extremity testing devices to simulate the actual work rather than the standard exercise test.

Although job simulation provides more specific assessment for some jobs than energy expenditure matching, results are limited by the artificial work environment of the testing lab. External influences and psychological possibilities must again be subjectively added to the analysis.

On-the-Job Monitoring

Either or both of the above work assessment methods will provide sufficient information to answer the return-to-work question for the majority of patients. In cases of unusual jobs and/or unusual work circumstances, accurate assessment may require on-the-job monitoring. Various ambulatory monitoring devices, such as portable 24-hour ECG recorders (see Chapter 14), make this kind of actual measurement possible.

In the real work setting, the pressures of an overzealous supervisor, an alcoholic coworker, intense heat, or impossible deadlines may produce responses that never could have been generated outside the work situation. A work diary is kept to correlate responses to circumstances. Once responses are identified, the question of patient's health and well-being in the same job or the need for a job change can be addressed.

To accomplish the on-the-job work assessment, a trial return to work may need to be arranged with the employer. The Phase III nurse may find one of her greatest challenges in educating employers in behalf of her patients.

(Patient ID Stamp)

C. P.

| | CARDIAC REHAB |
| | PROGRESS NOTES |

Date/Time	PROGRESS NOTES
5/20/XX 11 a.m.	Admission assessment:
	Patient discharged 5 days ago, after AMI on 5/1/XX.
	S. Patient and wife interviewed today prior to initiation of Phase III rehab program (see completed nursing history). Patient is eager to participate in anything that will help him "get things back to normal." Wife is supportive.
	O. Inpatient records reviewed. Transfer conference with N. S., R.N. on 5/16. After initial fear and anxiety, inpatient rehab progressed well. Physical condition remained stable throughout inpatient stay. Rehab objectives met, diet needs some follow-up. Heart rate limit for Phase III activities at 120 following predischarge EST.
	A. Ready to begin Phase III rehab. Has good knowledge base and is well motivated.
	P. Walking program to be initiated. Participation in Phase III group exercise and educational sessions to be scheduled. See Rehab Plan for summary of specifics.
	C. R. R.N.

(Patient ID Stamp)

C. P.

| | CARDIAC REHAB NURSING HISTORY |

Interview Date: 5/20/XX   **Preferred Name** "Nickname"
Age 42   **Sex** M   **Race** C   **Religion** Catholic
Education M.S. in Education   **Marital Status** Married 13 years
Significant Others Wife S. P., daughter G. P., son B. P.
Referring Physician D. D., M.D.
Occupation Teacher/Head of High School English Department
Place of Employment Regional High School

CARDIAC HISTORY:

On morning of 5/1/XX patient developed a cramping sensation in neck and jaw while feeding his cattle. He was lifting 5 gallon buckets of water when discomfort began and quickly radiated from neck and jaw to right shoulder and arm. He hurried to get animals taken care of before pain got worse. Patient then went into house and took aspirin and antacid to relieve pain and lay down on the sofa. Pain persisted for nearly 2 hours before patient called his family physician who instructed him to have his wife drive him to Community Hospital ER where he would have Dr. J. D. see him. Patient was diagnosed as having an acute inferior MI.

GENERAL STATE OF HEALTH:

Patient felt he had always been in good health, able to work long hours, and do heavy physical tasks.

REVIEW OF SYSTEMS:

Head—occasional frontal "sinus headaches," relieved by aspirin.
Eyes and Nose—no problems.
Respiratory—no problems.
Cardiovascular—since discharge has had occasional "muscular cramping" across chest with activities involving arms over head, relieved when activity ceases.
Skin, GI, GU, Metabolic—no subjective findings.
Allergies—none.
Medication—aspirin for headaches, occasional antacids for stomach discomfort, only past medications.

FAMILY HISTORY:

Mother—69, hypertension
Father—74, history of stroke, angina, and hypertension
Brothers—one died at age 45 of AMI (2 years ago), two others, one age 36 being treated for hypertension, the other, age 33, healthy.
Sisters—one age 38 healthy
Children—daughter age 9, son age 6, both healthy.

C. P.	**CARDIAC REHAB NURSING HISTORY**

PSYCHOSOCIAL:

Sleep/Relaxation—falls asleep O.K., frequently awakens with aching legs and hips, takes aspirin and Valium to get back to sleep; no specific time for or method of relaxation prior to MI.

Activities—works full time, farms part time, occasional fishing

Current Medications—has NTG 1/100 gr. for chest pain, has not taken any since discharge, has Valium 2 mg. for p.r.n. use, usually takes at bedtime.

Alcohol—none

Tobacco—quit smoking (cigarettes) 16 years ago.

Recent Losses—brother died suddenly 2 years ago, acute MI.

Financial—"no worse problems than anyone else."

Relationships—very close to wife and children; at present aunt is living with patient's family while uncle is in local hospital.

Usual Reactions—"get quiet and walk away" when angry, usually vents frustrations through physical farm work.

Sexual Status—resumed usual activities upon return home, denies difficulties.

Occupation—

Presently enjoying summer off from teaching; plans to resume part time in September; feels teaching job has a lot of stress and may "resign" from Department head position and "just teach." Has arranged assistance from friends and family for most of farm work. Plans to resume farming activities when physician gives the O.K., based on EST, etc.

SUMMARY:

See admission note; needs/problems identified on Rehab Plan.

C. R., R. N.

References

1. WATTS, R., "Sexuality and the Middle Aged Cardiac Patient," *Teaching and Rehabilitating the Cardiac Patient; Nursing Clinics of North America,* Vol. 11, No. 2, June 1976, pp. 349-459.

2. KELLERMAN, J. J., et al., "Return to Work After Myocardial Infarction," *Geriatrics,* March 1968, pp. 151-156.

3. WENGER, N. K., et al., "Uncomplicated Myocardial Infarction: Current Physician Practice in Patient Management," *JAMA,* Vol. 224. No. 511, 1973.

4. FOX, S. M., NAUGHTON, J. P., and GORMAN, P. A., "Physical Activity and Cardiovascular Health; Part III: The Exercise Prescription—Frequency and Type of Activity," *Modern Concepts of Cardiovascular Disease,* June 1972, Table 5.

5. ZOHMAN, I., and TOBIS, J., *Cardiac Rehabilitation* (New York: Grune & Stratton, 1970), p. 179.

13

planning of phase III cardiac rehabilitation

Behavioral Objectives

After completion of this chapter, the reader should be able to:

■ identify common nursing goals of Phase III.

■ describe at least two exercise approaches appropriate for patients during the early postdischarge period.

■ suggest three ways to strengthen patient self-esteem in Phase III.

■ discuss the nurse's role in vocational rehabilitation.

■ present objective guidelines that are useful in advising patients about return to sexual activity.

■ relate the importance of a thorough nutritional history.

■ recognize obesity as a behavior problem and develop a general plan for modification.

■ identify the five types of hyperlipidemia.

■ name two direct effects of smoking to be included in smoking education and four suggestions to ease the problem of smoking withdrawal.

■ state five common problems in long-term medication compliance and suggest preventive nursing actions for each.

■ recommend a plan for preparing the families of cardiac patients to handle future emergencies.

Introduction

Planning to reduce the trauma of transition from the protective hospital environment to the ever-changing pressures of the real world is the challenge facing the nurse specialist in the Phase III program. Table 13-1 presents common nursing goals used as guidelines in developing a Phase III rehab plan. The knowledge and skills needed to achieve these goals are discussed in the following pages.

Table 13-1
Common Nursing Goals of Phase III

Physiological

To assist the patient to return safely to his usual daily activities or to find acceptable substitutes for activities that are not appropriate.

Psychosocial

To help restore the patient's self-esteem by:
Accepting him as a person.
Including him as an equal partner on the health care team.
Providing a consistent professional contact for any questions, problems, or communication needs.
To assist the patient to reestablish his usual relationships at home, at work, and in society on a meaningful level.

Educational

To emphasize behavioral adjustments necessary for attainment of an optimal health state.

Planning to Meet Physiological Goals

Helping the patient to return to his usual level of activity or to find acceptable substitutes for activities that are contraindicated is a giant step toward the broader cardiac rehab goal of optimal physical health. While activities in Phase II helped prevent deconditioning, Phase III activities are designed to help the patient gradually regain strength and confidence. Since complete healing of the infarct area takes approximately six to eight weeks, major increases in heart rate prior to that time should be avoided. Phase III activities should be conducted well within the heart rate tolerance demonstrated during predischarge testing.

Three different types of activity can be planned in the immediate postdischarge period.

The At-Home Walking Program

The traditional posthospitalization exercise prescription is "a daily walk." The value of walking cannot be disputed. It is the most available, least costly, and for many, the most enjoyable form of exercise available. However, the classic instruction of "take a walk every day" leaves too much room for misinterpretation. Walking instructions need to be more specific.

The physician's order for at-home walking is written during discharge planning. The Phase II nurse provides basic instruction about the walking program to the patient and family before discharge. Follow-up responsibility to see that the patient understands his walking program and is performing it correctly belongs to the Phase III nurse.

Most people equate the success of any walking exercise with the greatest distance covered. In terms of caloric expenditure and weight loss, their thinking may be correct. In exercising cardiac patients, it is erroneous. Although distance can be used as a general reference, walking programs for cardiac patients are guided by heart rate response. Since the patient's heart rate limit has been established by testing, his walking program is constructed to keep his heart rate within the known limits.

Structured walking programs like the one outlined by the Colorado Heart Association[1] can be utilized, or a simplified program emphasizing heart rate response may be considered. A sample walking program is shown in Table 13-2.

The Phase III Low-Level Exercise Program

Where outpatient facilities are available, it is recommended that the patient be scheduled for a supervised, preferably monitored, exercise session once a week. Weekly exercise appointments accomplish two Phase III purposes. First, they provide opportunity for patient-nurse communication and second, they allow for frequent assessment of progress and adjustment of the health care plan.

Low-level exercises appropriate for Phase III patients can be planned in either of the following ways.

Group Cardiac Calisthenics. Calisthenics for cardiac patients must be carefully selected to avoid isometric contractions. Push-ups, pull-ups, sit-ups, and the like are inappropriate. "Cardiac calisthenics" is the popular term used to describe the isotonic and flexibility calisthenics recommended for cardiac patients. These exercises are easily carried out in outpatient programs using gym facilities and can be adapted to smaller groups in a monitored unit.

In the monitored unit, the number of patients per group will be limited to the number of monitor channels utilized. When possible, assignment to these smaller groups should be based on like capabilities.

In both locations, performance is guided by heart rate response, keeping the rate within each individual's limitations. A useful approach in conducting cardiac calisthenics is to start with exercises of the head and neck and work downward. Once the patient becomes familiar with the exercises, he will find the routine an easy one to do at home. Figure 13-1 displays some of the exercises that can be used. Workouts can begin with one minute per exercise at a leisurely pace. Time and pace can then be increased according to heart rate tolerances. Later, cardiac calisthenics can be used as warm-up exercises in Phase IV.

The group calisthenic approach allows for a special exercise adaptation—the participation of spouses in the calisthenic group. Of course, medical clearance, possibly including an exercise stress test, would need to be obtained for the spouse. Mutual involvement at this time would provide a psychological

Table 13-2
Phase III Walking Program

Week One After Discharge

Begin walking at a comfortable pace for five minutes. Then stop and rest (or leisurely stroll). Walk again (back to start) for five minutes.

Check your pulse periodically to be sure it is not too high. If your pulse is too high at any time, slow down or stop and rest. Try to walk a little faster each day, still doing five minutes at a time and being certain to keep your pulse within the prescribed limit.

Week Two After Discharge

Walk at a comfortable pace for ten minutes. Then stop and rest (or leisurely stroll). Walk again (back to start) for ten minutes.

Check your pulse periodically to be sure it is not too high. If your pulse is too high at any time, slow down or stop and rest. Try to walk a little faster each day, still doing ten minutes at a time and being certain to keep your pulse within the prescribed limit.

Week Three After Discharge

Increase walking time to 15 minutes.

Week Four After Discharge

Increase walking time to 20 minutes.

Week Five After Discharge

Increase walking time to 25 minutes.

Week Six After Discharge

Increase walking time to 30 minutes.

Weeks Seven and Eight

Maintain 30-minute walking periods (60-minute total). Increase walking speed, keeping heart rate within prescribed limit. Walking distance being covered will surprise you!

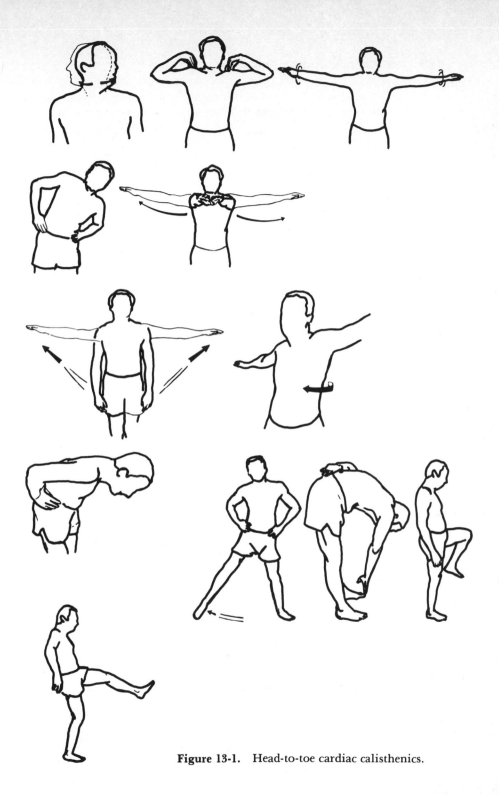

Figure 13-1. Head-to-toe cardiac calisthenics.

boost to the patient and a firsthand insight to the spouse. The encouragement given and the understanding gained through this exercise endeavor is likely to extend into other areas of the patient's rehabilitation program.

Low-Level Exercise Performance. In outpatient units equipped with various exercise appliances (discussed in detail in Chapter 18), patients in Phase III may be scheduled for individual exercise appointments using one or several of the devices at low levels, again guided by heart rate response. The treadmill can be easily used to simulate the patient's at-home walking program and, thus, provides a good performance assessment. For the more restricted patient or the one with a low-work tolerance, this individualized approach may allow closer monitoring and finer exercise adjustments than group calisthenics.

Exercise Precautions

Planning for Phase III activities implies concomitant planning for instructing the patient in the precautions to be observed when he undertakes his walking or calisthenics or any increase in daily activity at home. Table 13-3 lists major precautions to be covered with patients before Phase III exercise is started at home.

Table 13-3
General Exercise Precautions

Your pulse rate is your most important exercise guideline. Know how to take your exercise pulse. Know your prescribed exercise pulse limit.

If your pulse rate is excessive or if you experience any unusual sensations, slow down or stop and rest. If distress is severe or prolonged, request immediate help to the nearest hospital emergency room.

When exercising away from home, always tell someone where you're going and how long you expect to be. Do not exercise in isolated areas alone.

Do not exercise outdoors in extremes of heat, humidity, cold, or wind. Consider indoor alternatives such as enclosed climate-controlled shopping malls for walking or substitute cardiac calisthenics at home.

Exercise before eating or allow at least two hours to pass after a large meal before attempting exercise.

Avoid smoking before exercise.

Postpone exercise at times of strong emotion or fatigue.

Planning to Meet Psychosocial Goals

Rebuilding Self-Esteem

As discussed in Chapter 11, the loss of self-esteem that usually accompanies a heart attack may be profoundly felt by the patient returning home. The home environment is "normal," things are as they were. The patient is not the same, internally translated as "not normal." He is not able to instantly fulfill his usual roles and he begins to doubt that return to "normal" is even possible.

It is at this point that activation of therapeutic elements to strengthen self-esteem can be initiated through a Phase III program.

Activity Progression. Immediate involvement in a positive progressive activity program such as the one just described communicates to the patient that he is expected to improve. Patients begin to feel more comfortable and confident as they are able to demonstrate to themselves that a return to a "normal" and productive life is tangible self-evidence of progress that has a dramatic effect in helping the patient overcome feelings of depression and regain a sense of self-worth. Thus, provision of satisfactory exercise experiences in Phase III jointly contributes to physiological goals and psychological improvement. Through realization of his strengths and capabilities, the patient's fears of invalidism and worthlessness are negated.

Family Involvement. A critical step in rebuilding self-esteem is security in the love and acceptance of significant others. Involvement of the spouse (or other significant person) and family in rehab planning will provide mutual awareness of the patient's health status and goals and promote communication.

One of the greatest sources of contention that is apparent in families seems to result from patient and spouse having different understandings of the physician's orders.[2-3] This may be alleviated if patient and spouse receive the instructions jointly and are given written information and directions. If the patient and spouse both have a clear understanding of the disease, healing process, effect of diet, medications, and activity, they will be better prepared to make prudent decisions on their own regarding questions that arise during the first few days at home. Specific examples of family involvement are suggested throughout Unit III.

Professional Support. The simple fact that a busy, knowledgeable professional is willing to take the time to talk with the patient, answer his simple questions, and be sincerely concerned about his feelings dramatically enhances the patient's feeling of worth. Knowing that his nurse is available and when and how she can be contacted provides security at a much needed time. The influence of the nurse's attitude of acceptance and optimism should not be underestimated.

Peer Exchange. During hospitalization, the patient was isolated from his familiar groups: work group, social group, religious group, and so on. Until he again feels confident about himself physically and psychologically, he is likely to hesitate rekindling his group associations. But, the need for communication with others having like interests and concerns is intrinsic. And since the concern now of highest priority to the patient is his health state, involvement with others having the same priority will help the patient gain support, reassurance, and awareness that he is not isolated with his disease. Important peer pressure to comply with the suggestions of life-style modification that are essential to his health is a second advantage.

The Phase III group needs to be well planned so that therapeutic effectiveness is maintained. As group coordinator, the nurse should assess patient attitudes and personalities in scheduling group discussions. Although the open forum approach has its advantages, it is not necessarily the most appropriate for the early postdischarge patient who needs consistency and security. The group organized around like needs or problems is probably most functional for Phase III patients.

Group discussions among patients about their psychological reaction to their illness and its management are beneficial for both patient and staff. Staff members are better able to relate to the patients if they have a clear understanding of their attitudes and feelings, and the patients usually have a more positive attitude after they discover that their emotions have not been too unusual and that other patients have felt the same way.

Patients participating in such a group are best directed before the session to try to identify their feelings, to formulate in their own minds a statement which would describe some of their feelings about their disease and its influence on their life and the lives of those around them. Many times patients go through their recovery process feeling distressed, but not really taking the time to analyze their feelings.

Patient-spouse groups may be organized to help deal with feelings and emotions relating to the effect the cardiac event has had on their life and the lives of the other family members. They too should be directed to try to identify their feelings prior to coming to the group session.

Rebuilding Interpersonal Relationships

Interpersonal issues most directly affecting the postmyocardial infarction patient's psychological adjustment are work and sex. Although some educational groundwork has been laid for handling these issues in previous rehab phases, personal concern over lovemaking and working usually reaches its peak early in Phase III.

Health care planning for Phase III should anticipate these problems and provide for appropriate nursing intervention.

Return to Work. Vocational rehabilitation is defined as "an activity or service to train or retrain a client for employment and which pulls together all forces of the community." It assesses the strengths and weaknesses of an individual. The counseling relationship develops a rehabilitation prognosis and a rehabilitation plan to help return the cardiac client to his or her maximum capacity in the world of work.[4]

The Employed. It should not be assumed that because the patient is about to resume his previous job or a similar one, that his work-related problems are solved. Many practical problems arise in daily job situations that may be in direct conflict with the patient's efforts to follow his planned path to optimal health. Frustrating problems include arranging schedules to allow time and energy for exercise; ignoring the urge to start smoking again when others around take frequent "cigarette breaks"; maintaining a diet in the restaurant or cafeteria; remembering to take medication during a busy day; "keeping cool" at an emotionally charged meeting; not submitting to overwhelming deadlines and pressures.

The nurse should be prepared to discuss any of these problems with the patient and to provide realistic alternatives from which the patient can choose appropriate adjustments. Discussion with the employer or more specific intervention by another professional, such as the occupational therapist or vocational counselor, may be required.

The Retired. Being prepared to deal with retirement problems requires that the nurse be informed about the retirement circumstances. The patient near retirement age who voluntarily retires as a result of his cardiac disease presents one set of problems while the younger patient who is "forced" into retirement presents another.

In the former case, slower life-style may lead to boredom and depression. Planning should include assistance or resources to help the patient find a meaningful alternate to work. For example, the patient might enjoy the activity and status of being "recruitment chairman" for a newly organized cardiac club.

Forced retirement generally presents more complicated problems. In fact, the patient may be quite disabled. Medical restrictions may limit participation in the exercise program. Fear of sudden death and loss of control over life events may result in anxiety, anger, and a number of other defense reactions. Psychological counseling may be indicated.

The Unemployed. The obvious concern for patients who are not able or not allowed to return to work and are not eligible for retirement is financial. Realizing the loss of self-esteem experienced by a patient in this predicament, the nurse should be prepared to make referral for financial assistance and to request specific intervention of another professional, such as a social worker.

The nurse should also recognize that some patients may not want to return to work and will seek medical disability to gain a socially acceptable unemployment. Again, professional counseling may be necessary.

In assisting the patient in his vocational rehabilitation, then, the nurse functions as educator—of the patient, the family, and when necessary, the employer—, and professional liason—contacting other health professionals, such as vocational rehab counselors, occupational therapists, social workers, and psychologists.

Return to Sexual Activity

Most patients in Phase III will have the capability to resume sexual experiences, either on a preinfarction level or with some modification. Unfortunately, some patients and/or their spouses retain fears and misconceptions which act to deter sexual activity. Resumption of sexual activity should be discussed with the patient and spouse in explicit terms, providing accurate and specific information about the reestablishment of coitus and lovemaking in their lives.

A discussion of the assessment of sexual habits and attitudes was offered in Chapter 12. It bears repeating that it is essential that the discussion concerning resumption of sexual activity not be one-sided, with the health educator providing all the information. Information which only the patient and partner have will have a direct influence on the outcome of such a discussion. Their attitudes, beliefs, values, habits, and current emotional and psychological status are all factors which could interfere with resumption of normal sexual activity. Certain disease conditions, such as diabetes mellitus and neurological or genitourinary diseases, may prohibit physiological functions, as may drugs or alcohol abuse. Problems in these areas may require special intervention by sex counselors or medical treatment.

Hellerstein and Freidman state that "over 80 percent of post-coronary subjects can fulfill the physiologic demands of a majority of jobs and of sexual activity without symptoms or evidence of significant strain."[5] Their feeling is that most middle-aged cardiac patients who are not in congestive heart failure are capable of performing the sex act.

At it's peak, sexual intercourse has been assigned a five-to-six-MET value and patients who attain this level or higher on predischarge exercise testing should feel comfortable about returning to sexual activity on a level enjoyed prior to their illness.[6-7] It has also been demonstrated through indirect monitoring (ECG Holter recording rather than direct or photographic observation) with mature cardiac subjects, who have been married for a time and who engage in sexual activity in the privacy of their own home, that the heart rate response during intercourse averages less than 120 beats per minute and lasts for 10 to 15 seconds at most. The equivalent oxygen cost is similar to many other common activities, such as climbing a flight of stairs, walking briskly, and so on.[8]

Patients who have had a submaximal exercise stress test prior to hospital discharge have the advantage of having measured their physiological response to stress and can have this equated to either the MET requirement or the heart rate of less than 120 beats per minute. With this information, patients may feel more comfortable with their physical ability to tolerate sexual activity and, thus, have less psychological stress.

Patients who demonstrate significant signs and/or symptoms at levels lower than five METs should be advised to limit their activity to levels which will not cause symptoms. These patients and their spouses may need particular encouragement to participate in some type of sexual expression which is gratifying to both, yet not overtaxing to the cardiac partner. Discussions should be encouraged that will help them to identify their feelings about this development in their lives and their attitudes toward alternate expressions of love and methods of sexual gratification. They should understand the need of each person to be loved and accepted as he/she is. The couple may be helped by recalling signs of love each partner showed the other during courtship, such as the joy of simple caressing or of verbally expressing love. Forms of sexual expression both partners can enjoy may range from masturbation to gentle sexual intercourse with the cardiac patient restricting isometric muscular activity as much as possible. Oral or gentle manual stimulation might also be acceptable. Patients who exhibit a limited capacity to exercise at the beginning of Phase III should realize that recovery has just begun and that they may well return to significantly improved function after a period of reconditioning.

It is not unusual to experience a degree of deconditioning, even with a progressive inhospital activity program. This, coupled with the usual feelings of depression and physical weakness that occur when the patient first returns home and contemplates restructuring his life, is likely to have the effect of decreasing libido and/or sexual function. Patients who demonstrate the physical capacity of five METs, but who are distressed by the feelings of weakness and depression upon returning home may wish to return to sexual activity in a gradual manner, such as is suggested for the more debilitated patient.

General considerations for patients before they engage in sexual activity include the same considerations that are necessary prior to any type of activity at this stage of recovery: engaging in the activity when well rested, avoiding activity in extremes of temperature, humidity, or altitude, and waiting an hour or two after meals to become involved in an activity. In addition, the cardiac patient should consider the psychological implications and added stress of engaging in sexual activity in other than comfortable surroundings or with other than a familiar partner. Couples may find sexual activity is more enjoyable in the morning after a good night's sleep. Adequate time for a postcoital rest period should be allowed.

Alcohol consumption prior to sexual activity is inadvisable for the cardiac patient due to its vasodilatation effects and its tendency to increase heart rate. Alcohol may also affect the patient's perception of symptoms or his intellect in taking appropriate action in the event that symptoms do occur.

Patients who experience angina with sexual activity may find they can alleviate this symptom by the use of nitroglycerin prior to coitus.

Hellerstein and Freidman report that of patients in a physical fitness program, frequency and quality of sexual activity was reported improved in over 30 percent while being worsened in only 7 percent.[9] Thus, as the patient progresses through Phase III and into the Phase IV reconditioning program and approaches desired levels of fitness, he may look forward to sexual performance with greater satisfaction.

Planning to Meet Educational Goals

Throughout the rehab process, educational needs vary from patient to patient and educational planning is individualized. In Phase III, general educational emphasis is placed on aspects of life and health that affect psychosocial adaptation of the postmyocardial infarction patient and his family.

Dietary Changes

Eating is a social event having emotional, ethnic, and economic roots. Successful change in eating habits requires the combined insight and ingenuity of nurse, physician, dietitian, patient, and family.

Nutritional History. All dietary instruction is preceded by a comprehensive nutritional history. The nutritional history can be designed to follow the same outline as a basic nursing history (see Table 13-4). The information can be collected in conjunction with the initial outpatient interview, or a specific counseling session can be scheduled for this purpose.

Physical measurements are also useful in establishing a nutritional base. Anthropometry is the science of measuring the human body, its parts, and functional capacity. Measuring height and weight should be done routinely. Standard height-weight charts of normal ranges according to age can be used to classify the patient, but often can be misleading. The person who is overweight is not always obese. Large muscle mass, as in a weight lifter, will cause an increase in weight. Obesity, however, is the result of excessive body fat.

Table 13-4
Nutritional History

Medical Records Review

Has the patient followed a special diet previously? If so, for what reason?
What was his diagnosis?
Did he adhere to the diet?
Has he maintained the eating change?

Vital Statistics

Address (Is this a private home, hotel, apartment?)
Age (Will patient accept change?)
Sex (Who cooks the meals?)
Race (Are there cultural tastes that may affect adherence?)
Marital Status (Does patient live alone?)
Educational level (Will patient be able to understand a diet?)
Does he know basic nutrition—four basic food groups?
Occupation (Where and when will meals be eaten?)

General State of Health

What is usual and normal eating pattern?
Will a special diet be necessary?

Review of Systems

Visual or olfactory impairment will affect acceptance of foods.
Weight gain or loss—due to poor eating habits or disease process?
Medications—related to diet in any way?

Past Medical History

Is the patient allergic to any foods?
Has the patient a history of anorexia or overeating?

Family History

Were or are other family members over- or underweight?

Psychosocial

Summary of patient's life-style and self-concept.
Data obtained here may be the major factors determining adherence to a new eating plan.

Special skin fold calipers are available to determine the amount of subcutaneous fat in a person's body. Measurements are usually taken over the triceps and in the subscapular area. Men are considered obese if the triceps measurement is greater than 15 mm. and women if the measurement is greater than 25 mm.[10]

Therapeutic Diets. Most often, the nutritional needs of the cardiac rehab patient result from the presence of coronary risk factors. Several risk factors, including diabetes mellitus, hypertension, obesity, and elevated blood lipid levels can be partially or completely controlled by dietary adjustments. Hypertensive patients may be placed on a low-sodium diet with or without accompanying antihypertensive medication. Strict adherence to a specified ADA diet and the use of oral hypoglycemics or insulin will help control diabetes. *The Problem of Obesity.* As a risk factor, obesity can be controlled by having the patient change eating habits. The United States abounds with fad diets, fancy gadgets, and marvelous gimmicks, all gauranteed to shed those extra pounds in record time. None are successful in the long-term management of obesity. Professional assistance is needed to help guide the patient to lose weight realistically. Friendly encouragement by the nurse may be all one patient needs to stick to a prescribed regimen, while another patient will need psychological counseling.

Obesity is a complex problem that cannot be reversed overnight. One question which only the patient can answer is "why do I overeat?". Patterns of overeating are usually "inherited" based on a given culture. Types of foods, amount of servings, and frequency of meals are all carried over from generation to generation. These patterns are extremely difficult to change, and patients need much encouragement to incorporate prescribed diets into their particular life-style.

Because obesity is often an addictive state of complex conditioning, behavior modification may be recommended. Behavior modification is based on the assumption that if a certain behavior can be learned, it can be unlearned then redirected, or the learned behavior can simply be retrained. This approach with the obese patient as described by Williams[11] would follow these basic actions: identify specifically the problem behavior and the desired behavior; record baseline behavior and analyze; manage the situational forces surrounding the behavior; evaluate the present overall program. (Table 13-5 presents an application example.)

Enrollment in a weight reduction class gives many patients the peer recognition and acceptance to attain their desired weight. Caution is advised in considering group programs. Not all are appropriate for cardiac patients and some are health hazards, even for healthy individuals. The nurse should take the responsibility for reviewing and, if possible, visiting the program being considered to assure its usefulness to the patient. In all cases, medical permission should be obtained for the patient to participate.

Hyperlipidemia. Elevated lipid levels are a primary risk factor. Increases in plasma cholesterol and/or triglyceride have been linked to increased incidence of coronary disease.[12]

Table 13-5
Behavior Modification Approach to Obesity

1. Problem behavior	Overeating based on anxieties, that is, frustration, anger.
Desired behavior	To stop overeating when upset.
2. Record baseline behavior	Patient has high level of anxiety, becomes upset with coworkers and spouse. Pattern appears to be low-food intake beginning of week, but by Friday, high intake into the weekend in correlation with "pressures" on the job. Eating is highest at home in the evening.
3. Manage the situational forces	Evaluate "why" patient becomes upset—realistic anger? Avoid contact with foods—do not go to snack bar when angry. Do not keep ice cream in the freezer. Try to control upsets and outbursts of impulsive snacking by having a close friend monitor during the day. May need to eat more frequent meals with smaller portions. Keep a diary of intake and be honest. Eat meals slowly, never alone—have pleasant conversation with meal partner. Chew slowly, enjoy every bite. Provide reinforcement for positive behavior; if no snacks today, use the money that would've been spent on snacks for a nonedible treat (book, new jewelry, and so on.)
4. Evaluate	Objectively evaluate if approach is working; if not, find new approach.

Cholesterol and triglyceride levels should be obtained as a routine part of nutrition assessment to determine if a gross lipid abnormality exists. If either result is elevated, a more sophisticated blood study, lipoprotein electrophoresis may be indicated.

Cholesterol and triglycerids are water-insoluble lipids. Therefore, to facilitate transport throughout the body, these substances combine with protein. Depending on the amounts and types combined, different lipoproteins are formed. Electrophoresis identifies the lipoproteins present and helps classify the abnormality as a type (I through V) or hyperlipidemia.[13] Table 13-6 summarizes lipoprotein descriptions.

Table 13-6
Lipoprotein Classifications

Lipoprotein	Make up	Association	Risk of CAD	Function
Chylomicrons	60-95% Triglyceride/ cholesterol 5-40% Protein/ phospholipid	Hyperlipidemia Type: I, V	Elevations of chylomicrons does not seem to be associated with coronary risk at the present time.	Transport exogenous triglycerides
Prebeta or very low-density lipoprotein (VLDL)	60-80% Triglyceride/ cholesterol 20-40% Protein/ phospholipid	IV, V	The higher the VLDL level, the greater the risk for CAD.	Transport endogenous triglycerides
Beta or low-density lipoprotein (LDL)	45% Cholesterol 20% Phospholipid 25% Protein 10% Triglyceride	II, III	The higher the LDL level, the greater the risk for CAD.	Transport 1/2 - 3/4 of plasma cholesterol
Alpha or high-density lipoprotein (HDL)	50% Protein 15-30% Phospholipid 20-25% Cholesterol		Recent studies indicate that if HDL level is increased, the coronary risk is decreased.	Function not clear; may assist in transport of cholesterol.

Adapted from Herbert, P., *Hyperlipoproteinemia—A Return to the Basics* (Washington, D.C.: National Institutes of Health; 1977); LaRosa, J. C., "Dietary Therapy of Coronary Artery Disease," *Coronary Disease Learning System* (Denver, Colorado: International Medical Corp., 1974); Fredrickson, D., et al., *The Dietary Management of Hyperlipoproteinemia, A Handbook for Physicians and Dieticians* (Washington, D.C.: National Institutes of Health, DHEW Pub. No. (NIH) 76-110, 1974); Gotto, A. W., "Recognition and Management of the Hyperlipoproteinemias," *Heart and Lung*, July-August 1972, pp. 508-518; and Medical News, "High Blood Lipid Levels," *JAMA*, Vol. 237, No. 11, March 14, 1977, pp. 1066-1067.

A separate dietary plan has been prepared by the National Institute of Health for each of the types I through V of hyperlipoproteinemia. The corresponding booklet can be taken home for use as a guideline for eating adjustments following review and discussion of the appropriate plan with the patient and family.

High-Cholesterol Levels. The patient with a moderately increased cholesterol level may be advised to follow a prudent diet as outlined by the American Heart Association.[14] The prudent diet emphasizes a decrease in saturated fats. In fact, a prudent diet may be generally prescribed for postmyocardial infarction patients. Together with a moderate reduction in caloric intake, this less complicated dietary adjustment can contribute tremendously to improved nutritional health.

General Nutritional Counseling. The therapeutic diets reviewed in the preceding section are based on specific health problems. Dietary interventions described require a physician's order. It should be noted that the effectiveness of strict dietary prescriptions is still uncertain.[15]

In the interest of progressing toward optimal health, the nurse specialist in Phase III can initiate general nutritional counseling for patients and families not needing a therapeutic diet. A review of the basic four food groups and the amounts needed to maintain a sound body is a healthful reminder to everyone from time to time. General advice to reduce common dietary excesses may be offered in the hope of improving nutrition (see Table 13-7).

Educational Approaches. There are many objectives a patient and nurse may agree upon in planning achievement of the prescribed diet. To help the patient reach his goals, the nurse might consider the following:

1. Leading a discussion of the objectives in a group composed of patient, spouse, and dietitian.
2. Arranging for the dietitian to instruct the patient and spouse, giving cognitive information regarding the diet management and implementation.
3. Developing affect by leading discussions in the exercise group among patients on similar diets; providing tasty recipes and menus; frequently inquiring about the enjoyment of the diet, method of food preparation, and demonstrating interest in its implementation; arranging for a buffet supper where each party would bring a covered dish appropriately labeled (low cholesterol, low salt, and so on) and the recipe so members could taste new dishes. This could be followed by an educational program presented by a dietitian.
4. Evaluating psychomotor ability by discussions with patient and spouse regarding food preparative methods, label reading, and menu planning.

In the preceding examples, a dietitian, a nurse, and other patients were included in the educational team. Dietary education can be successfully carried out through a number of educational approaches: one-to-one counseling, family group teaching, large patient groups, and so on. A combination of approaches may help provide the motivation needed for the patient to effect dietary change.

Table 13-7
Toward Healthful Eating

Reduce intake of	Increase intake of
Alcohol	Fish
Caffeine beverages (coffee, tea, cola)	Fresh fruit
Calories (decrease quantities of food)	Poultry
Red meats	Roughage (grain, raw vegetables)
Refined carbohydrates	Water (at least eight glasses per day)
Salt	
Saturated fats (replace butter with vegetable oil)	

Special Considerations:

Five to six small meals per day may be more healthful than three larger ones. Eating in a relaxed manner with pleasant company aids digestion. Vigorous activity should be curtailed until at least two hours after eating.

Cessation of Smoking

Smoking, like obesity, is essentially a behavior problem. Unlike obesity, however, the deleterious effects of smoking are rarely tangible. The problems created by smoking are well publicized, but seldom taken personally.

Facts. The first step toward cessation of smoking is awareness—awareness that smoking *is* a problem. Statistics relating cigarette smoking to lung cancer, emphysema, bronchitis, peptic ulcer, oral cancer, and coronary artery disease, though impressive, are not likely to strike a note of caution. However, facts about the direct effects of cigarette smoking on the patient may have more personal impact. Two specific actions should be explained and applied to the patient.

Nicotine Effects. FACT: Nicotine is a chemical stimulent causing a temporary "high," and over a period of time, biological dependency.

PERSONAL CONSIDERATION: Some patients rely on cigarettes to ease tension during a busy day or to help them unwind in the evening. Are you in this category?

FACT: Because of its stimulant property, nicotine acts on the central nervous system to increase the amount of adrenalin released in the body. In turn, heart rate, blood pressure, and cardiac output increase. In the cardiac patient, these increased demands on cardiac function may result in poor work-activity tolerance, chest discomfort, shortness of breath, or serious rhythm abnormalities.

PERSONAL CONSIDERATION: Think what walking up a flight of stairs while smoking a cigarette will do to your heart! Have you ever had a similar experience?

Carbon Monoxide Effects. FACT: Burning tobacco produces carbon monoxide. The carbon monoxide in cigarette smoke when inhaled enters the bloodstream and attaches itsélf to red blood cells, reducing the ability of those cells to carry oxygen. When an increase in activity takes place and the heart demands an increased supply of oxygen, the blood will not be able to deliver. Again, the result will be some symptom of cardiac distress.

PERSONAL CONSIDERATION: Compare heart rate responses before smoking a cigarette, while smoking but not inhaling, and while smoking and inhaling.

Approaches. If the patient has no desire to stop smoking, any "no smoking" campaign will be fruitless. It is hoped that educating the patient concerning cigarette hazards will generate added motivation to quit. Emphasis should be placed on the fact that many negative effects of smoking can be reversed regardless of how long the patient has been a smoker. "I've been smoking for 40 years, it won't do me any good to quit now" is not defensible.

Books, pamphlets, films, and in some locations, counselors are available through the American Heart Association, the American Lung Association, and the American Cancer Society—all valuable resources for kicking the habit. An increasing number of group programs are available through community agencies, church-affiliated groups, and proprietary organizations. Health care personnel can provide valuable models for patients. Nurses who continue to smoke while advising their patients to quit are poor examples of personal commitment to health and fitness. Table 13-8 presents additional tips on smoking cessation.

Medication Compliance

Taking medications when and how they are prescribed is important to the health, and frequently even the life, of the cardiac patient. Every patient should have a thorough understanding of his medication as related to his disease, not just an awareness of isolated drug facts. The patient's understanding of his medications should be evaluated periodically and updated when necessary.

Table 13-8
Helpful Hints to Stop Smoking

Most people can't identify *why* they smoke. A diary of *when* may provide some insight. Professional counseling may aid self-analysis.

Most people cannot stop "cold turkey." Gradual weaning will help reduce the physiological withdrawal symptoms—tremors, palpitations, irritability, sweating, and so on.

Most people will not be successful if others close to them continue to smoke. Husband and wife should consider quitting together.

Most people are not successful in changing more than one behavior at a time. Obese smokers may do better to stop smoking first, then begin dietary changes.

Most people initially need a substitute behavior for smoking. Instead of having a cigarette, do something harmless—drink a glass of water, nibble on carrots or celery, chew on flavored toothpicks, eat sugarless mints, and so on.

Most people don't realize the cost of their smoking. Start a "dream fund" and during withdrawal save the money that would have been spent on cigarettes. When you've successfully quite for six weeks, reward yourself!

Chapter 8 described the initial objectives and general data of comprehensive drug education. These guidelines are equally appropriate during Phase III and throughout the patient's health care. No nurse should be satisfied with telling a patient just once about his drugs. Until compliance has been evidenced in the patient's usual environment, drug education is incomplete.

The need for medication may change as the patient progresses. With a good knowledge of his medications, the patient will be better able to describe to his physician signs or symptoms which may indicate a need for medication adjustment. Improving physical condition may decrease the need for such drugs as tranquilizers, antihypertensives, antiarrhythmics, diuretics, hypoglycemics, antihyperlipidemia agents, and long-acting nitrates. Conversely, some medications will affect the ability of the patient to exercise safely. Adrenergics fall into this category as do many over-the-counter cold remedies (see Chapter 17).

Jinks states that factors promoting medication noncompliance include chronic illness requiring long-term maintenance; advanced age; lack of continuous follow-up by a single physician; and a large number of medications.[16] Other authors add financial problems to this list.[17-18] Unfortunately, most cardiac patients have one, a combination of, or all of these factors to contend with.

To enhance compliance, Phase III nursing should include the following:

- reevaluating the patient's knowledge, compliance, and drug effects at frequent intervals;

- offering frequent encouragement to continue the medication regimen;

- teaching comparison shopping techniques, or obtaining prices for certain cardiac medications from several local pharmacies and offering a comparison list for the patient;

- checking that elderly patients, those with poor eyesight or arthritis of the hands can manage their medications; for example, can the patient read the labels on the bottle or is the typing too small? Can the patient open the childproof lid? Is there someone available to help remind those whose memories are poor to take their medication?

- providing a method by which the patient will be able to manage a medication regimen which requires taking a large number of medications accurately. For example, a daily checklist of the medications and times each is to be taken; a series of bottles marked with the medication times for putting the day's supply of pills in the proper container each morning. The local pharmacist may be able to suggest products available to use in helping to remind the patient to take the medications at the proper time and in the proper amounts.

- suggesting to patients who attend a clinic, or are treated by a physician group and have the problem of not being followed by a single physician, that they take a list of all their current medications for the physician's review each time they visit the office. They should also be encouraged to speak freely with the doctor about medications and make sure they have all their questions answered to their satisfaction.

Emergency Education for Families

The family, of course, should be involved in all Phase III teaching. Dietary changes and smoking cessation are best achieved through joint effort. Reminders about medications from family members may help prevent complications.

Educational planning in Phase III should also address a family problem that tends to arise when the patient returns home: "What will we do if it happens again?" "How will we know if it's another heart attack?" Early in Phase III, the patient and family should be taught:

- how to recognize a heart attack. Table 13-9 is a sample handout to reinforce teaching.
- how to summon emergency assistance; entry into the community's emergency medical services system should be planned in advance; emergency phone numbers should be taped on every telephone in the patient's home; the quickest route to the nearest emergency room should be identified.
- what to do until help arrives; the American Heart Association recommends that all families of cardiac patients be taught basic life support, starting with teaching fifth graders mouth-to-mouth resuscitation techniques and eighth graders closed chest massage.[19] Cardiac patients themselves should be instructed in CPR performance. Contrary to common belief, patients are not jeopardized by the physical exertion of resuscitation. In fact, patient's responses monitored during mannikin practice stayed well within their prescribed activity limit.[20]
- remembering that the first two hours after a heart attack hold the greatest risk of death, it is of utmost importance that the patient and family be encouraged not to delay seeking medical attention if a heart attack is suspected. A teaching program for all family members with use of a mannikin can be arranged in coordination with the local Heart Association. All cardiac rehab nurses should be certified instructors in cardiopulmonary resuscitation.

Recognizing the usual needs of patients and families in Phase III, knowing the treatment alternatives available, and having identified the patient's specific problems through nursing history, it remains for the Phase III nurse to work with the patient in assembling the pieces into a coherent Phase III cardiac rehab plan. Steps in solving problems and achieving rehab goals should be presented in the form of behavioral objectives. Time frames expressed in objectives should be realistic and conservative.

Once drafted to the satisfaction of patient and nurse, communicated to other health professionals on the rehab team, and documented on the patient's chart, the Phase III rehab plan is put into action. The following sample case illustrates the results of Phase III planning.

Table 13-9
Heart Attack: What to Look for/What to Do

Most Common Symptoms

Chest pain
Prolonged crushing pain in the center of the chest
Squeezing discomfort or heavy ache in the center of the chest

Radiation of pain
Pain may act like "stomach trouble"
Pain may "travel" to arms, neck, shoulder, back or jaw

Accompanying Symptoms

Nausea
Vomiting
Sweating
Shortness of breath
Feeling of weakness
Palpations

What to Do

Stop activities
Sit down or lie down
If the pain lasts longer than two minutes

Call your doctor
Phone number _____
If your doctor is not *immediately* available, arrange for most prompt mode of transport

Ambulance phone number _____
Tell dispatcher you think you are having a heart attack.
Private car
Upon arrival at emergency room, report to main desk and inform personnel you think you are having a heart attack.

(Patient ID Stamp) C. P.			CARDIAC REHAB CARE PLAN	
Date Identified	Need/Problem	Approach	Behavioral Objectives	Date Achieved Changed
5/20/XX	**Physiological**		The patient will be able to	
	1. gradually advance toward resuming usual	1. a) implement Phase III at home walking	1. conduct a progressive walking program at home keeping heart rate well	
	daily activities 2. begin to promote "exercise habit"	program 2. b) schedule for monitored	within prescribed limit and without any negative effects, as evidenced by	
		cardiac cal. group once/wk.	the patient's verbal reports and home exercise record.	
			2. express interest in consistent exercise performance verbally and through	
			group attendance	
	Psychosocial			
	3. very anxious to	3. a) re-emphasize	3. accept the need for	
	"get back to normal," may tend to overdo	importance of gradual activity resumption	gradual activity increases as evidenced by performing within limitations	
		b) check frequently re activities	assigned during Phase III	
		being done at home c) discuss slow		
		but sure return to normal with		
		wife, encourage her helping patient		
		monitor extent of activities		

(Patient ID Stamp) C. P.			CARDIAC REHAB CARE PLAN	
Date Identified	**Need/Problem**	**Approach**	**Behavioral Objectives**	**Date Achieved Changed**
	4. concern of too	4. encourage	The patient will be able to 4. by end of Phase III,	
	much stress at work	discussion of work alterna- tives, i.e.	reach a decision re return to former teaching posi- tion in the fall	
		stepping down from department head position,		
	Educational	farming full time, etc.		
	6. continue diet education (low cholesterol)	6. a) schedule counseling session to	6. implement low cholesterol diet successfully as indicated by discussion	
		get complete nutritional history	of correct meals, recipe suggestions, etc.	
		b) encourage discussion with other		
		patients on same diet c) have dietitian		
		provide summer recipe ideas		
		d) invite patient and wife to attend next		
		group session on diets.		

(Patient ID Stamp) C. P.			CARDIAC REHAB CARE PLAN	
Date Identified	Need/Problem	Approach	Behavioral Objectives	Date Achieved Changed
	7. review	7. a) emphasize that	The patient will be able to 7. a) eliminate or modify arm	
	a) types of exercise b) use of NTG	most arms-above-head activities are	activities that have been causing chest dis-comfort	
		isometric and explain physiology;	b) use NTG correctly for chest discomfort	
		discuss activities involved		
		b) have patient explain when NTG is indi-		
		cated and how it should be taken, stored,		
		etc.		

(Patient ID Stamp)

| C. P. | PHYSICIANS' ORDER SHEET |

Date/Time	ORDERS
5/14/XX 9 a.m.	Schedule to begin as out-patient next week.
	Use heart rate of 120 for Phase III activities.
	Diet: low cholesterol
	Meds· NTG 1/100 gr. p.r.n. for pain
	Valium 2 mg. p.r.n. for restlessness.
	J.D., M.D.

References

1. CARDIAC RECONDITIONING AND WORK EVALUATION UNIT, *Exercise Equivalents* (Denver, Colorado: Colorado Heart Association, 1970), p. 23.
2. WISHNIE, H. A., HACKETT, T. P. and CASSEM, N. H., "Psychological Hazards of Convalescence Following MI," *JAMA* Vol. 215, No. 8, 1971, pp. 1292-1296.
3. HAMBURG, D., HACKETT, T. P. (consultants), *Coping with Cardiovascular Disease*, (Nutley, New Jersey: Hoffmann-LaRoche Inc., 1974).
4. GEHRKE, A., "Vocational Rehabilitation of the Cardiac Patient," *Cardiac Rehabilitation*, Vol. 6, No. 4, Winter 1976 (New York: American Heart Association, New York State Affiliate), p. 31.
5. HELLERSTEIN, H. K. and FRIEDMAN, E. H., "Sexual Activity and the Post-coronary Patient," *Medical Aspects of Human Sexuality*, March 1969.
6. WATTS, R., "Sexuality and the Middle-Aged Cardiac Patient," *Teaching and Rehabilitating the Cardiac Patient; Nursing Clinics of North America* (Philadelphia: W. B. Saunders Company, Vol. 2, June 1976), pp. 349-459.
7. HELLERSTEIN, H. K. and FRIEDMAN E. H., "Sexual Activity After a Heart Attack," *Primary Cardiology*, October 1975.
8. *Ibid.*
9. *Ibid.*
10. MAYER, J. "Obesity: Diagnosis," *Postgraduate Medicine*, Vol. 25, No. 469, April 1959.
11. WILLIAMS, S. R., *Nutrition and Diet Therapy*, 3rd ed. (St. Louis, Missouri: The C. V. Mosby Company, 1977), p. 511.
12. MEDICAL NEWS, "Experts Link Heart Disease and Diet," *JAMA*, Vol. 237, No. 24, June 13, 1977, p. 2593.
13. FREDRICKSON, *op. cit.*
14. ESHLEMAN, R. and WINSTON, M., *American Heart Association Cookbook* (New York: David McKay Company, Inc., 1975).
15. MANN, G. V., "Challenging Some Sacrosanct Beliefs About Diet and Nutrition," *Resident and Staff Physician*, March 1977, pp. 88-95.
16. JINKS, M., "The Hospital Pharmacist in an Interdisciplinary Inpatient Teaching Program," *American Journal of Hospital Pharmacists*, Vol. 31, June 1974, pp. 569-573.
17. STORLIE, F., *Patient Teaching in Critical Care* (New York: Appleton-Century-Crofts, 1975).
18. GENTRY, W. D. and WILLIAMS, R. B., *Psychological Aspects of Myocardial Infarction and Coronary Care* (St. Louis, Missouri: The C. V. Mosby Company, 1975).
19. AMERICAN HEART ASSOCIATION and NATIONAL ACADEMY of SCIENCES—NATIONAL RESEARCH COUNCIL, "Standards for Cardiopulmonary Resuscitation and Emergency Cardiac Care," *JAMA Supplement*, February 1974, p. 850.
20. ABBOTT, R. A., et al., "Cardiopulmonary Resuscitation Training for Cardiac Patients in Exercise Programs," *Heart and Lung*, September-October 1978, pp. 829-833.

14

implementation of phase III cardiac rehabilitation

Behavioral Objectives

After completion of this chapter, the reader should be able to:

- arrange a Phase III schedule appropriate to his/her health care setting.
- give at least six examples of intranursing referrals useful in Phase III.
- describe in some detail the components of emergency preparation in an outpatient cardiac rehab setting.
- illustrate electrode placement for two common telemetry leads used in monitoring exercise.
- perform a satisfactory skin prep to precede exercise monitoring.
- identify at least six common causes of motion artifact seen during exercise monitoring.
- explain the use of Holter monitoring in Phase III rehab.

Introduction

Having assessed the postdischarge patient's health status and having formulated a rehab plan based on the results of that assessment, the Phase III nurse's next step is action. Putting the plan into action assumes that attention has already been given to operational details affecting implementation. How should the program be structured? What equipment and supplies are needed? And how will progress be followed?

Program Methods

The structure of the Phase III cardiac rehab program depends upon institutional policies, physical facilities, and medical opinion. However, the biggest influence on the Phase III design is the nursing emphasis placed on the importance of this rehab segment. Phase III nursing services can be implemented by several methods.

The Informal Phase III Program

In many hospitals, nurses have carried out selected Phase III functions throught the existing hospital system. That is, they have followed the patients after discharge through cardiology clinics, or where permitted, direct hospital-to-home telephone contact. Both of these methods provide an opportunity for communication and problem solving. However, the lack of planned continuity is frustrating for the patient ("Will you be calling every week at the same time?" "Can I call you anytime?") and the lack of total services is frustrating to the nurse ("If only *someone* could talk to his boss . . . ." "Mrs. Jones would be less worried if she could talk with other patients' wives.").

The informal approach can be improved upon by arranging "postdischarge nursing appointments." Patients and families could return to the hospital to meet with the nurse at scheduled times. All that is needed is a small conference room and a policy supporting this much needed nursing follow-up. Most goals of a Phase III rehab plan could be met through several such visits complemented by group educational programs.

The Formal Phase III Program

A Phase III program conducted as the first half of a comprehensive outpatient cardiac rehab program provides the ideal location for postdischarge follow-up. The outpatient rehab unit becomes the hub of all the patient's rehab activities. The place and the people quickly grow familiar and provide the patient with security.

For most patients, a once-a-week exercise appointment is satisfactory to check progress. The number and frequency of educational sessions will depend upon the patient's/family's learning and counseling needs. Table 14-1 displays several scheduling approaches and presents the major advantages of each.

Table 14-1
Phase III Scheduling Approaches

Plan I	Plan 2
Daily walking at home Weekly monitored exercise appointment	Daily walking at home Weekly monitored exercise appointment
Phase III patients scheduled Tuesday or Thursday Cardiac calisthenics in groups of four	Phase III patients intermingled with Phase IV patients, appointments anytime Low-level exercise appliances
Weekly group educational programs	Monthly group educational programs
Every Wednesday evening For patients and families Rotation of standard Phase III topics (for example, diet, sex, smoking, activities, stress, and so on) every six weeks	Combined programs for Phase III and Phase IV patients Topics selected according to general group need Individualized teaching done nurse-to-patient in conjunction with exercise visits
Specific counseling sessions by appointment.	Specific counseling sessions by appointment.
Advantage: Emphasizes Phase III problems and needs; promotes individual attention.	Advantage: Combined approach may provide added psychological boost and enhance long-term motivation. (Phase IV patients provide models of successful rehab.)

Plan 3	Plan 4
Daily walking at home	Daily walking at home
Weekly exercise appointment	Monthly monitored exercise appointments
One evening per week in community gym facility Large Phase III group (including spouses where allowable) Unmonitored, but closely supervised	Weekly phone check on progress Visits scheduled more often if any problem suspected
Group education discussion session to follow exercise	Monthly group educational programs
Brief educational presentation Miscellaneous questions/ answers for group discussion	Schedule extra time before or after group for individualized instruction as needed
Specific counseling sessions by appointment.	Specific counseling sessions by appointment.
Advantage: Added peer support and encouragement from larger larger group; social involvement may enhance motivation.	Advantage: Provides basic Phase III services for patients having problems (distance, means of transportation, finances) that limit more frequent participation.

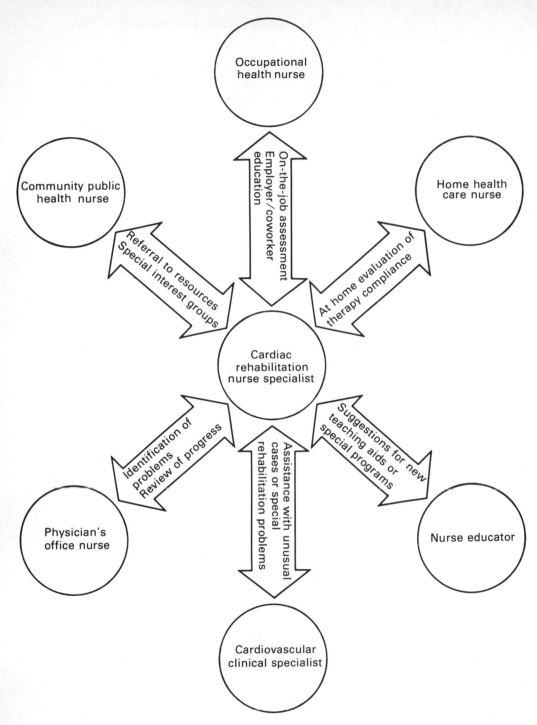

Figure 14-1. Nursing network for Phase III rehabilitation.

The Collegial Network

Regardless of how formal or informal the Phase III program may be, patient services can be greatly enhanced through utilization of a "nursing network for rehab." To explain, the Phase III nurse specialist or the primary care nurse in a Phase III role is in the position to request nursing advise and/or assistance from many valuable nursing colleagues. Nurse-to-nurse consultation, one of the most underused rehab resources, can be the Phase III nurse's most valuable asset. Calling upon the knowledge and expertise of her peers to complement her nursing care provides the patient with the best professional care. Figure 14-1 illustrates how various nurses' services may be solicited to expand Phase III nursing coverage.

Program Mechanics

Emergency Preparedness

As the professional in charge of the outpatient cardiac rehab service, the nurse is responsible for the general welfare of all patients seen in any rehab program context. Of paramount concern in the outpatient cardiac rehab setting, as in any cardiac care area, is the possibility of cardiac emergency (see Chapter 19 for a detailed discussion of outpatient emergencies and complications). Inpatient locations of Phase I and Phase II programs automatically include coverage by an emergency plan. Since patients are first seen as outpatients in Phase III, implementation of Phase III rehab requires prior emergency preparation.

When organizing a Phase III program, the nurse assumes responsibility for assuring that emergency policies have been completed, that emergency equipment is functional, and that personnel are proficient in emergency procedures. The emergency plan must be totally operational before any patient is seen. Once completed, the emergency plan covers all Phase III and Phase IV outpatient functions.

Exact specifications for emergency preparation are a matter of institutional policy. The established emergency procedure of the CCU may be applied to programs located within hospitals, since the same coronary care committee may have jurisdiction over both areas. If the outpatient program is located in a community facility, specific step-by-step emergency actions will have to be identified.

The American Heart Association has defined minimum acceptable emergency preparation for outpatient rehab facilities:

> Emergency equipment, including equipment for cardiac resuscitation, should be available and should include defibrillators and emergency airway and ventilation equipment, as well as an array of drugs useful during cardiac emergencies. It is also desirable ... that an ECG machine be available. Personnel should be trained and certified in the principles and applications of cardiopulmonary resuscitation according to the standards published by the American Heart Association and the National Acadamy of Sciences—National Research Council.[1]

Table 14-2
Considerations for Emergency Preparedness in an Outpatient Cardiac Rehab Setting

Personnel	Equipment	Communication	Policies
Required	Crash Cart to include:	Inhouse notification systems:	To define responsibilities
Basic life support (BLS) training for all health professionals involved with the rehab unit	Airway and ventilation equipment IV solutions and supplies Medications	General alarm Direct page Special phone line	To state specific actions (including "standing orders")
Suggested	Oxygen supply and administration devices	Emergency medical services (ambulance) notification Phone numbers taped to each phone in unit	To document preparation and emergency readiness
BLS training for ancillary staff members; advanced life support training and CPR instructor certification for cardiac rehab nurses	Defibrillator Portable Self-contained oscilloscope (strip recorder desirable) Both line and battery power	Predefined emergency travel route	

The emergency cart or "crash cart" is a standard component of emergency equipment in cardiac care areas. Structure and composition of emergency carts vary somewhat with geographical location and institutional policies, but the basic components listed in the American Heart Association statement must be available.

In addition to equipment and supplies, emergency preparation requires development of a written emergency plan. The plan must specify the roles of each health care worker in the rehab unit. An effective communication system must be prepared, such as an emergency page number or an alarm. Advance planning for patient transfer—how, by whom, to where— is essential. If the rehab unit is in a community facility, the local ambulance service should visit the facility so that details such as accessible entrance and exits, elevator or stairs for fastest transport, and so on can be coordinated. Preparedness will save precious minutes, and it is hoped, precious lives, in the event that a rare emergency does occur. Table 14-2 summarizes emergency considerations.

Phase III ECG Monitoring

Determination of planning effectiveness is a nursing responsibility inherent in implementation. Were the treatment choices appropriate? Are the prescribed guidelines being adhered to? Is the plan working as intended? Objective data about success of the Phase III plan or need for change in terms of cardiac responses can be obtained through use of either telemetry monitoring or ambulatory ECG recordings. In some cases, complementary use of both observation techniques is most beneficial.

Monitoring is primarily employed in Phase III to guide program progress. A potential secondary benefit of both direct ECG observation via telemetry and indirect ECG monitoring via tape recording is the possible identification of postmyocardial infarction patients having rhythm abnormalities associated with increased risk of sudden death.[2] Complex ventricular ectopic activity, repetitive, multifocal, early-cycle ectopics, or greater than one ectopic per minute, over a period of time is a major forecaster of life-threatening events.[3] Identification of high risk patients during Phase III implementation may allow time for appropriate medical intervention and, thus, prevent cardiac crises.

Telemetry Monitoring. Outpatient cardiac rehab programs may or may not incorporate ECG monitoring systems (see Chapter 18). The availability of monitoring equipment for use with Phase III exercise provides the advantage of direct assessment of heart rate and ECG responses to exercise during this early postdischarge period.

Telemetry, the transmission of the ECG signal via radio frequency, is the ideal method for monitoring outpatient exercise sessions both in Phase III and in Phase IV. The use of telemetry combines freedom of movement for exercise performance with quick and easy application. The ECG clarity is excellent when motion artifact is controlled and lead selection is appropriate.

Lead Selection. Telemetry systems are bipolar. That is, they enable monitoring of one ECG lead whose vector direction is determined by the placement of the negative and positive electrodes. The bipolar leads most popular for use in exercise monitoring are those whose ECG presentation is most similar to V_5, the most sensitive ECG position for recording ST segment changes.[4]

Two of the more common leads monitored by telemetry during exercise are CM5[5] and CC5[6] Electrode placement for these bipolar chest leads is illustrated in Figure 14-2. Both leads place the positive chest electrode in the standard V_5 position. Figure 14-3 shows a side-by-side comparison of the two lead presentations.

Skin Preparation. Meticulous skin prep is equally as important to effective telemetry transmission as good lead selection. Skin prep requires shaving of the electrode sites, cleaning the areas with acetone or alcohol, removing the horny layer of epidermis by brisk rubbing with rough gauze or fine sandpaper. Each step contributes to improved impulse conduction.

Once acquainted with the telemetry apparatus, the patient can be taught to do his own skin prep. Giving the patient responsibility for this important "hook-up" procedure conveys professional confidence in his ability to be independent, a Phase III psychological boost. Figure 14-4 is a sample of hook-up instructions that could be mounted adjacent to a mirror in the patient dressing area. A "prep tray" including electrodes, razors, acetone or alcohol swabs, and gauze or sandpaper could be arranged on a shelf or counter top beneath the mirror.

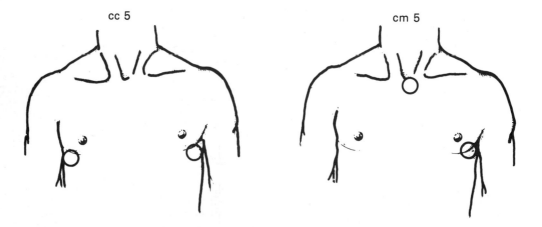

Figure 14-2.   Electrode placement for bipolar telemetry leads. (Left) Negative electrode placed in the fifth intercostal space, right anterior axillary line. Positive electrode placed in the standard V_5 position. (Right) Negative electrode placed on the manubrium. Positive electrode in the standard V_5 position.

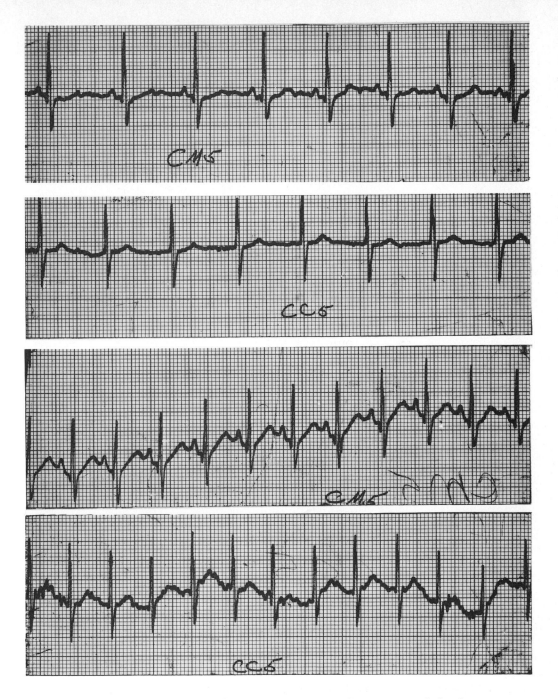

Figure 14-3. Telemetry lead comparison. The top two strips were recorded prior to exercise, the bottom two during exercise.

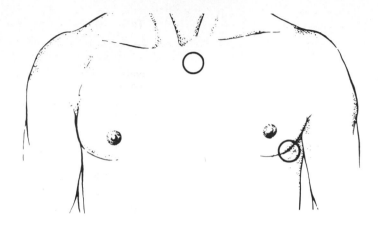

Figure 14-4. "Hookup" instructions. The circled areas are the sites where the electrodes should be placed. 1. Shave areas of all visible hair. 2. Wipe the areas with acetone. 3. Rub the areas with a gauze pad until they are red. 4. Apply electrodes to skin. 5. Attach transmitter and secure.

Electrodes. Most telemetry systems are adaptable to either disposable or reuseable electrodes. Disposables are "quick and easy," being applied to the prepared skin in one step. Reuseable electrodes require application of electrode paste and adhesive collars, a few extra steps for the patient to perform. However, the lower cost of reuseable electrodes may be well worth the few added minutes of time. In either case, silver/silver chloride electrode composition is desirable for the best conduction.

Reduction of Motion Interference. One additional concern that can render telemetry transmissions unreadable in spite of the best lead choice, skin prep, and electrodes is motion artifact. When motion interference appears on the monitor, a quick determination should be made as to the cause and corrective action taken. Some of the more common causes of motion artifact are listed in Table 14-3.

Ambulatory ECG Monitoring. Portable tape recordings of ECG activity, commonly referred to as "Holter monitoring" after Norman Holter, who perfected the system in the 1950s,[7] provide another technical means of following responses during implementation of a Phase III rehab plan. Recorders are available with reel-to-reel or cassette tape, 12- or 24-hour recording capacity and one or two ECG leads.

Use of a Holter monitor is technically similar to application of telemetry, requiring the same fastidious skin prep, similar lead placement, and attention to stabilizing lead wires to reduce motion. Most recorders are lightweight, the size of a pocket calculator and can be carried unnoticed in a cameralike case or attached to a belt.

Table 14-3
Common Causes of Motion Artifact During Telemetry Exercise Monitoring

Problem	Solution
Breast motion	Forewarn females to wear secure bras; modify electrode placement as necessary.
Electrode sliding	Remove excess electrode paste or replace electrode.
Electrode wire swaying	Secure loose wires with tape or elastic bandage.
Electrode wire tension	Make small stress loops taped close to electrode to reduce tugging.
Fatty tissue motion	Modify electrode placement in flabby subjects.
Lead wire problems	
Loose connections with disposable electrodes	Use of spring clips assures tight grips; snaps wear with use.
Broken lead wires with reusable electrodes	Have a spare replacement set available.
Muscle tremor	Check for isometric contraction, such as gripping; advise muscle relaxation.
Shivering	Check room temperature; suggest additional exercise clothing.
Transmitter bouncing	Secure transmitter in pouch holder, with belt clip, or with elastic bandage.

Useful throughout the cardiac rehab process, Holter monitoring allows documentation of cardiac responses in a variety of settings and situations where direct telemetry transmission is not practical or where professional observation would slant response findings. Effects of environment, psychological state, or unusual activities can be recorded in their natural habitat. Considered a diagnostic study, Holter monitoring requires a physician's order.

One disadvantage of Holter monitoring is the time lag from recording to documentation of results. Like any taped message, the tape must be played back for its contents to be analyzed. In retrospect, recorded results are correlated with events that are documented in a diary kept by the patient during the recording period. Table 14-4 lists specific Phase III uses of Holter monitoring. Figure 14-5 is an example.

Records and Reports

Records of performance and documentation of progress are required in this early outpatient program just as they are in all rehab phases. Outpatient forms can be designed to accommodate reporting either Phase III or Phase IV results as illustrated by the sample case at the end of this chapter.

Table 14-4
Phase III Applications of Ambulatory ECG Monitoring

Periodic Holters to assess Phase III progress

Recordings at predetermined intervals, such as every four weeks on all patients who had serious dysrhythmias during their acute course

Recordings on all patients midway through Phase III program, approximately three to four weeks postdischarge

Initial Holters to establish response baselines on patients in Phase III exercise programs without telemetry monitoring. Follow-up Holters for comparison when response questions arise during group of home exercise

Holters to determine responses in complex psychosocial situations

Actual on-the-job responses
Responses to sexual activity
Responses to special social events, such as attending a high school football game with son at quarterback or attending the company's annual formal dinner-dance
Responses to driving (or taking public transportation)

Holters to determine responses to unusual or questionable activities

Barbecuing, picnicing
Motorcycle or snowmobile riding
Playing chess or backgammon
Small animal care (chickens, pigeons, goats, dogs, and so on)

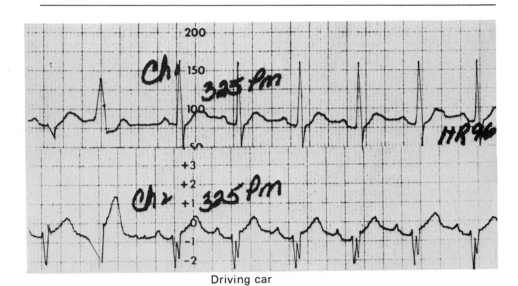

Driving car

Figure 14-5. Holter-recording excerpts. The following strips were selected from a 24-hour Holter recording to demonstrate the usefulness of long-term ambulatory monitoring in obtaining Phase III information: Two channels of ECG data were recorded: channel 1—modified V_5 chest lead; channel 2—modified V_1 chest lead. Strips are marked with the time of recording and respective heart rates. Corresponding activities were identified from patient diary entries. The recording ran from 3 P.M. one day to 3 P.M. the next.

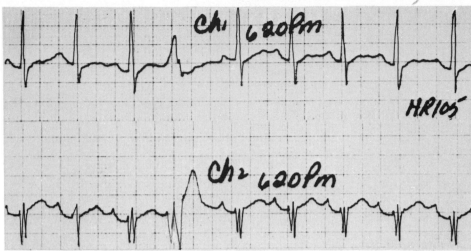

Hoeing flower bed

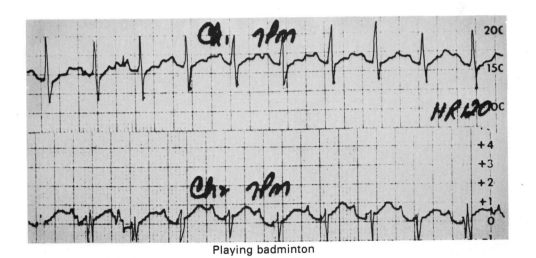

Playing badminton

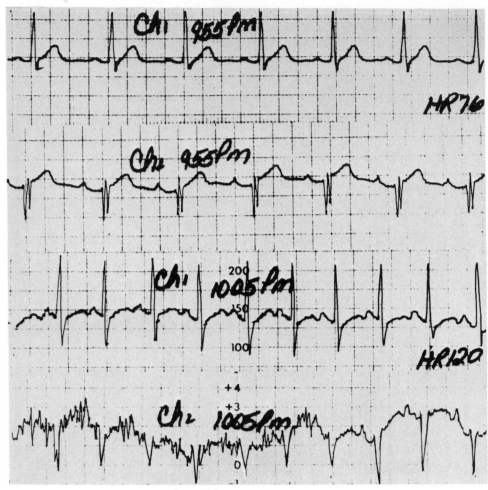

Sexual intercourse

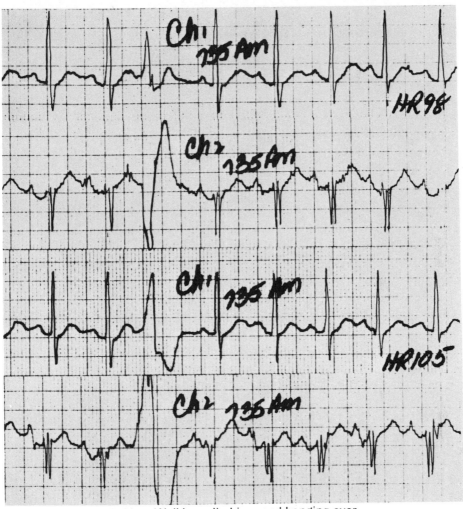

Working: Walking, climbing, and bending over

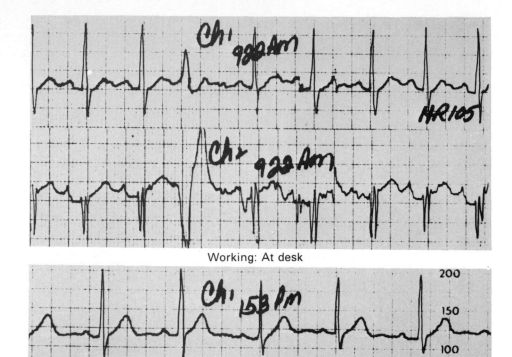

Working: At desk

At home: Resting and
having cold drink, "tired."

(Patient ID Stamp)

C. P.

**CARDIAC REHAB
PROGRESS NOTES**

Date/Time	PROGRESS NOTES
5/22/XX 9:30 a.m.	First Phase III monitored exercise session. Cardiac calisthenics performed by group of 4 patients led by nurse.
	S. Was enthused by group participation, talking and joking with other patients. Reports walking program initiated yesterday. Walked 10 minutes total, rested halfway. HR 90-96. No new occurrence of chest discomfort.
	O. First calisthenic session performed without difficulty. Rhythm remained stable. Responses as on therapy sheet. Performed exercises easily, no evidence of strain or fatigue. Shown how to put on telemetry electrodes.
	A. New activity seems to have provided needed boost to patient. Is tolerating low-level activities well.
	P. Patient advised to progress home walking per Phase III schedule. Scheduled same group appointment for next Thursday. Suggested that wife come along to observe. Nutritional review session to be scheduled to immediately follow.
	C. R., R. N.

CARDIAC EXERCISE THERAPY FLOW SHEET

Name   C. P.   Phase   III

Date/Time	Pre-exercise					
5/22/XX 9 a.m.	HR 76	Rhythm NSR	BP 124/86	**Device** **Load**	1 cardiac cals.	2
Program Week 1	**HR Guide** 120 limit		**Rx Date** 5/14/XX	**Time** **HR peak**	10 min. 104	
5/29/XX 9 a.m.	HR 82	Rhythm NSR	BP 124/78	**Device** **Load**	1 cardiac cals.	2
Program Week 2	**HR Guide** 120 limit		**Rx Date** 5/14/XX	**Time** **HR peak**	15 min. 94	
	HR	Rhythm	BP	**Device** **Load**	1	2
Program Week	**HR Guide**		**Rx Date**	**Time** **HR peak**		
	HR	Rhythm	BP	**Device** **Load**	1	2
Program Week	**HR Guide**		**Rx Date**	**Time** **HR peak**		
	HR	Rhythm	BP	**Device** **Load**	1	2
Program Week	**HR Guide**		**Rx Date**	**Time** **HR peak**		
	HR	Rhythm	BP	**Device** **Load**	1	2
Program Week	**HR Guide**		**Rx Date**	**Time** **HR peak**		

Physician _____ *J. D.*

Exercise Intervals				Post-exercise		
3	4	5	6	HR 82	Rhythm NSR	BP 122/80
				Total Time 10 min.	Supervised By *C. P., R. n.*	
3	4	5	6	HR 75	Rhythm NSR	BP 120/80
				Total Time 15 min.	Supervised By *C. R., R. n.*	
3	4	5	6	HR	Rhythm	BP
				Total Time	Supervised By	
3	4	5	6	HR	Rhythm	BP
				Total Time	Supervised By	
3	4	5	6	HR	Rhythm	BP
				Total Time	Supervised By	
3	4	5	6	HR	Rhythm	BP
				Total Time	Supervised By	

(Patient ID Stamp)	
C. P.	**NUTRITIONAL HISTORY**

Date 5/29/XX   **Interview with** ___C. P. and wife___

                                           By ___C. R., R.N.___

Medical Record Review:

Past medical records indicate no special diet prior to MI. Other than CAD, no medical problems requiring dietary adjustment. Currently prescribed a low cholesterol diet.

Vital Statistics and Nutritional Background:

Patient owns a farm property on which he lives with his wife and 2 school-aged children. Patient and wife feel the family eats a well-balanced diet, mostly homegrown vegetables and meats from the farm. The patient's wife does most of the cooking.

The patient normally eats a large breakfast (bacon, eggs, toast with butter, etc.) between a.m. feeding of the livestock and going to school. At school, he eats lunch in the cafeteria. The family eats a large dinner meal each evening, e.g. roast beef, mashed potatoes with gravy, fresh peas, salad.

Both patient and wife have a good understanding of basic nutrition and what foods are good for health. No predominant cultural influence on eating.

Review of Systems:

No known food allergies. No recent changes in weight. Weight has always been within normal range. No GI difficulties. Current meds (NTG and Valium p.r.n.) have no dietary influence.

Family History:

No unusual eating habits or weight problems in immediate family. Patient and wife receptive to adopting low cholesterol diet as family standard as long as "not too extreme."

Psychosocial:

Farming is the patient's preferred life-style. Farm animals include chickens (for eggs), steers (for beef), and pigs (for pork and bacon). Fresh vegetables are a specialty.

Summary:

S.   Have good basic understanding of adjustments needed for low cholesterol maintenance from diet education in hospital, "no butter, only 3 eggs a week, low fat milk, etc." But feel they need more specific suggestions. "There must be more to it."

O.   Dietary modifications will need to be consistent with family's usual food sources (e.g. unrealistic to advise patient to eat more fish than meat!). Type of beef, number of eggs, etc. will have to be discussed. Poultry and vegetables can be emphasized.

A.   Need more specific ideas and applications.

P.   It was recommended that patient keep a food "diary" next week of what foods and how much. Next dietary session will be scheduled with dietitian (approx. 2 weeks) to more specifically suggest modifications.

C. R. R.n.

References

1. COMMITTEE on EXERCISE, *Exercise Testing and Training of Individuals with Heart Disease or at High Risk for Its Development: A Handbook for Physicians* (New York: American Heart Association, 1975), p. 27.
2. DeBUSK, R. F., "The Role of Ambulatory Monitoring in Postinfarction Patients," *Heart and Lung*, July-August 1975, pp. 555-561.
3. LOWN, B. and WOLF, M., "Approaches to Sudden Death from Coronary Heart Disease," *Circulation*, July 1971, pp. 130-140.
4. BLACKBURN, H, et al., "Standardization of the Exercise Electrocardiogram," *Physical Activity and the Heart* (Springfield, Illinois: Charles C Thomas, 1967), pp. 101-133.
5. *Ibid.*
6. FROELICHER, V., et al., "A Comparison of Two Bipolar Exercise Electrocardiographic Leads to Lead V_5," *Chest*, Vol. 70, No. 5, November 1976, pp. 611-616.
7. "From a Frog's Muscle to Ambulatory ECGs," *Patient Care*, December 1976, p. 10, (Editorial).

15

evaluation of phase III cardiac rehabilitation

Behavioral Objectives

After completion of this chapter, the reader should be able to:

- describe at least two methods useful in evaluating a patient's psychosocial adaptation during Phase III.
- name two objective measurements that can be used to evaluate Phase III effectiveness.
- list at least six patient outcomes to be expected from an effective Phase III program.

Introduction

The duration of a Phase III rehab program generally coincides with the estimated time for healing, six to eight weeks after infarction. Assuming no new problems have arisen during this early postdischarge period, the patient should be ready to perform a near-maximal exercise stress test, the opening scene of Phase IV rehab. Relay of the patient from Phase III to Phase IV is a quiet event, blending evaluation of Phase III accomplishments with assessment of Phase IV needs.

Evaluation of Patient Responses

Phase III nursing emphasis has been on the need for psychosocial adjustments that result from altered health status due to an acute cardiac event. Every effort was made to reinstate the patient into his preferred life-style. Where return to previous habits would perpetuate health deficiency, modifications were suggested in an attempt to alleviate problems without having to reverse the patient's life direction. Extensive change in or total abstinence from, the patient's desired way of life is a last-resort effort to protect health.

Evaluation and summarization of Phase III achievements precede initiation of the more highly structured Phase IV outpatient program.

Subjective Evaluation

The patient's impression of progress, always difficult to measure, is the most useful index, in evaluating psychosocial adaptation. To add some form and consistency to subjective evaluation of Phase III effectiveness, several areas of personal response should be observed.

Behavior and Body Language. Patient behavior and body language are best evaluated over a period of time. Patients who enjoy a positive psychological outlook generally present themselves as self-assured, confident, congenial and carry themselves in an upright posture with "a bounce to their step." On the other hand, psychologically depressed cardiac patients present as less confident and content, and their entire appearance tends to droop: shoulders may hunch, facial muscles may relax or sag, and gait may be slow or even dragging.

Evaluation of such behavior over a period of time can clearly indicate to the nurse that the patient either is or is not approaching an optimal psychological state. Certainly everyone has trying days when he/she may appear to be psychologically depressed, and it is for this very reason that a nursing judgment should not be made upon an occasional observance. The judgment should be formulated from several different observations with the average behavior response being given the most weight.

Acceptance of Treatment Plan. The patient's attitude toward his disease and treatment plan can be a good indicator of his psychological state. In general, patients who are able to cope with their disease and diligently go about the business of adapting their life habits to improve their health demonstrate a more healthy psychological state. The patient who retains a strong element of denial of his disease finds himself in a quandary regarding behavioral changes and seems to present a more vacillating psychological state, usually requiring professional counseling.

Self-Evaluation Statements. Specific individual discussion or casual remarks in a group setting may convey the patient's perception of his own psychological state. Expressions of self-confidence and optimism obviously reflect an improved self-concept.

As part of the subjective evaluation, each patient should be specifically asked what fears or concerns remain to be resolved. Assurance can then be offered that specific attention will be placed on these problems as the patient continues his rehab progress into Phase IV.

Social Observations. Family discussions can help round out the subjective evaluation. How do family members perceive the patient's affect in various home situations? Anecdotes about the patient in his home environment will help confirm improvement or degeneration in psychological state.

Toward the end of Phase III, a conference should be scheduled to include all members of the rehab team who participated in the patient's Phase III rehab care. The conference provides a forum for sharing information and observations helpful in finalizing evaluation of the patient's psychosocial state.

Documentation of the nurse's evaluation of the patient's psychosocial state at the end of Phase III should include reference to the subjective information obtained. Findings that influenced the conclusion should be noted—observable patient behavior, attitude, self-evaluation comments, or other sources of information.

Objective Evaluation

As discussed in Chapter 14, assessment of physiological responses can be carried out through telemetry or ambulatory monitoring. Comparison of cardiac responses at the beginning and end of Phase III may supply demonstrable evidence of Phase III effectiveness. More specific data will, of course, be obtained from exercise testing (see Chapter 17). Comparison of initial Phase IV test results to predischarge test results may be the best objective reflection of Phase III effectiveness.

Formal psychological testing as an objective parameter of psychological status has been used in some rehab programs. On a routine basis, the value of such testing is limited since one-time administration of the more popular personality tests will not document attitude or personality changes.[1]

Expected Patient Outcomes

What can be expected of the majority of postmyocardial infarction patients at the end of Phase III can be expressed as common patient outcomes (see Table 15-1). Such a listing provides a general reference for measuring achievements by use of some of the methods just described. Each patient's rehab plan includes, of course, his individualized Phase III objectives. Accomplishment of stated objectives is the outcome desired for all cardiac rehab patients.

Table 15-1
Common Patient Outcomes of Phase III Cardiac Rehabilitation

Physiological Outcomes

Upon completion of the Phase III outpatient program, the cardiac patient should be able to:

Perform his usual daily activities, including work, sex, and low-level recreational activities, without difficulty, OR modify daily activities to an acceptable level on which they can be carried out safely and comfortably.

Carry out a daily low-level exercise program guided by prescribed responses.

Psychosocial Outcomes

Upon completion of the Phase III outpatient program, the cardiac patient should be able to:

Spontaneously display increasing self-confidence and optimism.

Express resolution to pursue more healthful life habits.

Demonstrate progress in re-establishing usual relationships.

Communicate life areas where fears or concerns remain.

Educational Outcomes

Upon completion of the Phase III outpatient program, the cardiac patient should be able to:

Demonstrate an understanding of his prescribed diet by describing dietary adjustments he has made.

Discuss personal negative effects of smoking and indicate a desire to cut down or quit (or already have done so).

Describe signs and symptoms of a heart attack and relate a plan-of-action for handling a cardiac emergency.

Transfer Considerations

Since there is no change in physical location, the transfer from Phase III to Phase IV is a more dramatic event on paper than it is in action. What is observable is that an outpatient visit in one week is for Phase III exercise and in the next week it is for an exercise stress test. Before and between these visits, discussions, reviews, and analyses complete Phase III evaluation and transfer.

(Patient ID Stamp)

C. P.	**CARDIAC REHAB** **PROGRESS NOTES**

Date/Time	PROGRESS NOTES
7/6/XX 9 a.m.	Patient to be transferred to Phase IV program. Initial EST scheduled for 7/11.
	Phase III rehab summary:
	Objectives achieved as noted on Rehab Plan, although tendency to overdo
	should be frequently re-assessed.
	S. In the last 2-3 weeks, patient has been increasingly anxious to do more.
	Frequently reminded not to overdo. States he feels "good" and enjoys
	both walking program and monitored sessions.
	Has had no recurrence of chest discomfort experienced during first few
	days after discharge.
	O. Has carried out walking program appropriately by monitoring heart rate
	response. Monitored sessions show stable rhythm with exercise at low
	levels. No excessive heart rate or B/P response. No undue fatigue or
	muscular strain resulting from calisthenics.
	A. More than ready to progress to Phase IV!
	P. EST scheduled for 7/11 a.m. Reviewed pretest instructions with patient.
	Scheduled for lab and x-ray.
	C.R., R.N.

References

1. Bruhn, J., "Obtaining and Interpreting Psychosocial Data in Studies of Coronary Heart Disease," *Exercise Testing and Exercise Training in Coronary Heart Disease* (New York: Academic Press, 1973), pp. 263-273.

unit IV

phase IV
cardiac
rehabilitation

16

background and basics of phase IV cardiac rehabilitation

Behavioral Objectives

After completion of this chapter, the reader should be able to:

- state the purpose of a Phase IV cardiac rehab program.
- identify specialized areas of knowledge and skill required in Phase IV nursing.
- outline normal physiological adaptations to exercise.
- define cardiovascular fitness.
- list at least ten contraindications to exercise and explain the underlying problem of each.
- list at least ten benefits of exercise and discuss the specific advantage of each for the cardiac patient.

Introduction

Each phase of the cardiac rehabilitation process has the ultimate goal of achieving the optimal health levels stated in the cardiac rehab definition. Built upon health care efforts during hospitalization and the immediate post-discharge period, Phase IV is the period during which rehab fulfillment will most likely be witnessed.

Purpose

Health care emphasis in Phase IV is on secondary prevention. Attention is focused on developing healthful habits in the hope that recurrence of an acute event will be prevented. In some areas of concern about behavior like diet and smoking, changes have already commenced. Phase IV will offer the patient the support and reassurance to persist.

The predominant health dimension in Phase IV is exercise. Exercise testing and exercise training occupy much of the time and effort of both patients and professionals in Phase IV.

Unlike the three preceding phases, Phase IV is not demarcated by physical events. No transfer or discharge signals its start. Instead, initiation of Phase IV depends upon the rate of physiological recovery of the myocardium from its acute injury. Since scar formation occurs at different rates in different patients, the point at which patients enter Phase IV will vary based on the physician's evaluation of readiness. Most patients begin Phase IV between six to twelve weeks after their acute event.

Nursing Requisites

Nursing continuity is necessary throughout the total rehab process. Therefore, nursing functions in Phase IV are continuous with those in Phase III. The addition of exercise as a major treatment element should be an outgrowth of previous health teaching and discussion.

To effectively carry out the nursing process, the nurse specialist in Phase IV must add to her expertise the knowledge and skills related to exercise as a diagnostic study, as a therapeutic intervention, and as a desirable way of life. Table 16-1 provides an overview of specialized Phase IV nursing requirements. Succeeding chapters discuss nursing functions in detail.

One additional consideration for the professional nurse practicing in Phase IV deserves mention—personal fitness. As in any health care setting, patients and families look to professionals to be role models. If patients are expected to learn, accept, and practice exercise as a life habit, the nurse must be ready, willing, and able to practice what she preaches.

Exercise Physiology: The Basics

An understanding of the changes that occur in body functions as a result of exercise is essential to effective Phase IV nursing. Exercise physiology is an emerging science. The purpose here is to acquaint the nurse with the basic

Table 16-1
Specialized Nursing Requirements for Phase IV Cardiac Rehabilitation

Cognitive	Psychomotor
Basic exercise physiology	Operation of exercise stress-testing equipment
Exercise indications/contraindications	Monitoring/recording equipment
Exercise stress testing	Testing apparatus
Principles and purposes	Bicycle ergometer
Methods, modes, protocols	Treadmill
Normal and abnormal responses	Operation of exercise-training devices and monitoring equipment
Resting and exercise ECG assessment	Performance of exercise routines
Exercise training	
Prescription development	
Training methods	
Home alternatives	
Long-term motivation	
Evaluation of exercise responses	
Improvement indicators	
Problems and complications	

concepts forming the foundation for the exercise-testing and training approaches to be presented.

Oxygen and Exercise

The key to understanding exercise physiology is a thorough knowledge of the oxygen transport mechanism. When dealing with exercise, two facets of oxygen transport must be considered.

Systemic Oxygen Transport. The normal oxygen transport sequence was reviewed in Chapter 6. Recall that in a resting state, oxygen is distributed in the body according to certain homeostatic priorities. The brain, the heart, and the kidneys get first priority of circulatory flow and oxygen delivery. Should some pathology interfere with this order, the body will make all adjustments possible to re-establish the priorities.

Exercise Adaptations. A shift in homeostatic priorities occurs in an exercise state. The brain and the heart maintain first and second positions respectively, but third priority is now redirected to the skeletal muscles actively performing the exercise. Since skeletal muscles are a low priority on the distribution list during rest, the increased flow to this large system during exercise must be supplied from other systems not as active at the time. In fact, the kidneys and the gastrointestinal tract operate on near minimal circulatory flow during exercise so that high-volume flow can be provided through vasodilatation to the third exercise priority—skeletal muscles.

This process of defining and supplying homeostatic priorities from rest to exercise is called circulatory redistribution or "preferential shunting."[1]

The second major oxygen transport adaptation during exercise occurs at the extraction level. The amount of oxygen diffusing from the blood (hemoglobin) to the cellular mitochondria of skeletal muscle greatly increases in response to the added supply needed to perform the exercise. Evidence of this adaptation can be readily observed if the venous oxygen content at rest is compared to the venous oxygen content during exercise. The latter result will be much lower. Skeletal muscle has the ability to increase oxygen extraction from the arterial blood supply as much as three times during exercise. These arterial-venous oxygen changes and others that occur in the oxygen transport cycle with exercise are outlined in Table 16-2. Assuming that all oxygen transport mechanisms are intact and that circulatory redistribution occurs as predicted, an individual will usually be able to exercise to a high level of physical work. If some abnormality limits either transport or adaptation, the work performance tends to be low grade.

Maximal Oxygen Uptake. There is a point during exercise at which the oxygen transport system is performing at peak efficiency, when all homeostatic adjustments possible have been made in response to the exercise stress. This top performance level is called the "maximal oxygen uptake."

> Maximal oxygen uptake is the greatest amount of oxygen a person can take in during physical work and is a measure of his maximal capacity to transport oxygen to the tissues of the body. It is an index to maximal cardiovascular function, provided pulmonary function and ambient oxygen concentration are normal and, therefore, is valuable in the evaluation of abnormal cardiovascular function.[2]

Table 16-2
Basic Physiological Adaptations to Exercise

	Rest	Exercise
Respiratory volume	5-8 L. of air per minute	Increases, as much as twelve times; both rate and depth of respiration increase
Cardiac output	5-6 L. of blood per minute	Increases, as much as four times; both heart rate and stroke volume increases
Arterial-venous oxygen content difference	5 ml. of oxygen per 100 ml. of blood	Increases, as much as three times; working muscle cells extract more oxygen

Adapted from Morehouse, L. and Miller, A., "Circulatory Adjustments During Exercise," *Physiology of Exercise* (St. Louis, Missouri: The C. V. Mosby Company, 1971), p. 123; Buskirk, E. R., "Cardiovascular Adaptation to Physical Effort in Healthy Men," *Exercise Testing and Exercise Training in Coronary Heart Disease* (New York: Academic Press, 1973), pp. 23-30; and Phillips, R., "The Biochemistry and Physiology of Exercise," *Medical Aspects of Exercise Testing and Training* (New York: Intercontinental Medical Book Corporation, 1973), pp. 13-18.

Since maximal oxygen uptake reflects efficiency of the total oxygen transport system, it depends upon maximal function of all adaptive transport mechanisms. In this regard, the near linear relationship between maximal heart rate and maximal oxygen intake proves useful in evaluating exercise test results and preparing exercise prescriptions. This will be discussed in subsequent chapters.

Maximal oxygen uptake is symbolized as max VO_2 (maximal volume of oxygen) and is usually expressed as milliliters per kilogram of body weight per minute of time. For example, a world class athlete may exhibit a max VO_2 of 75 ml. per Kg. per minute, a cardiac rehab patient with training 35 ml. per Kg. per minute, and a cardiac rehab nurse (without a personal exercise program) 25 ml. per Kg. per minute!

Oxygen transport measurements are made in research laboratories through use of cumbersome, mechanical respiratory analysis devices, or more recently by costly, sophisticated computerized units. In a cardiac rehab setting, neither approach is very practical. Fortunately, research results have been incorporated into conversion tables and activity lists that can be used in the everyday rehab environment.

Myocardial Oxygen Transport.   Awareness of the oxygen delivery system to the heart itself and of the influences on oxygen need in the myocardium is the next step toward understanding exercise in the cardiac patient.

There are three main determinants of myocardial oxygen need:[3]
1. Heart rate. The more frequently the heart contracts, the more oxygen is required.
2. Systolic blood pressure. The greater the left ventricular tension, the more pressure and oxygen are required for contraction.
3. Contractility. The greater the speed of contraction, the more oxygen is required.

Myocardial oxygen uptake is symbolized as MVO_2 (myocardial volume of oxygen).

Coronary arteries are the only route of oxygen transport to the myocardium. Because of continuous cardiac performance, the myocardium constantly extracts high levels of oxygen from coronary circulation. Little "extra" oxygen supply is returned to the coronary sinus.

When a demand for increased oxygen occurs, such as one or a combination of the preceding, this limited reserve does not become the major adaptive mechanism in the myocardium that the larger reserve is in skeletal muscle. In other words, the increase in oxygen extraction results in only a minor change in the arterial-venous oxygen difference in the myocardium as compared to the three-fold increase described as a transport adaptation in skeletal muscle.

The *remaining mechanism* for increased oxygen delivery to the myocardium is *increased flow through the coronary arteries.* This increased flow is mainly supplied by the increase in cardiac output resulting from both increased stroke volume and increased heart rate.

However, in patients with coronary artery disease, the degree of effectiveness of this delivery system depends upon coronary artery patency. If the increased flow is impeded by the poor condition of coronary arteries, the

Table 16-3

Contraindications to Exercise Performance

Interference with Oxygen Transport	Potential for Complications	Limited Performance
Left ventricular inadequacy (pump failure, congestive heart failure)	Acute MI	Musculoskeletal, neuromuscular, or arthritic disorders
Uncontrolled dysrhythmia (tachy-arrhythmia, A-V blocks, conduction defects)	Aneurysm (dissecting aortic, ventricular)	Alcoholism
	Embolism (pulmonary or systemic)	
Uncorrected valve disease	Phlebitis	Psychoses
Ventricular aneurysm	Uncontrolled hypertension	Marked obesity
Cardiomegaly	Infectious or febrile systemic disease	
Fixed rate pacemaker	Unstable angina (progressive, preinfarction angina, coronary insufficiency)	
Severe anemia	Uncontrolled metabolic disease (diabetes, hyperthyroidism)	
Myocarditis or pericarditis	Electrolyte disturbances	

Adapted from American College of Sports Medicine, *Guidelines for Graded Exercise Testing and Exercise Prescription* (Philadelphia: Lea & Febiger, 1975), pp. 10-11; Committee on Exercise, *Exercise Testing and Training of Individuals With Heart Disease or at High Risk for Its Development: A Handbook for Physicians* (New York: American Heart Association, 1975), p. 41; and Wenger, N. K., *Coronary Care: Rehabilitation After Myocardial Infarction* (New York: American Heart Association, 1973), p. 17.

myocardium will not receive the needed oxygen and myocardial ischemia will result. Such ischemia is usually evidenced by the occurrence of an indicative sign or symptom when the patient exercises.

Transport of oxygen to the myocardium cannot be measured noninvasively. Clinically, an index of myocardial oxygen delivery can be calculated by multiplying the heart rate at a selected exercise level by the systolic blood pressure at the same level. The result is known as the "double product," an approximation of the myocardial oxygen requirement.[4]

Cardiovascular Fitness

"Physical fitness," though currently in vogue, escapes precise definition. It means different things to different people; thus, discussions about this desirable state tend to take place in completely subjective terms. To lend some form to a nebulous concept, the President's Council on Physical Fitness and Sports offers this definition: "Fitness is the ability to carry out daily tasks with vigor and alertness, without undue fatigue, and with ample energy to enjoy leisure-time pursuits and to meet unforeseen emergencies."[5]

Cardiac rehabilitation deals with an even more specific idea of fitness— cardiovascular efficiency. Assuming concurrent efficiency in the pulmonary system, cardiovascular fitness represents optimal oxygen transport to perform daily activities comfortably, and the adaptability to readily increase the oxygen supply in times of stress.

The process of developing this level of fitness is known as "conditioning." The conditioning agent is exercise. Exercise training as carried out in the Phase IV cardiac rehab setting is, therefore, synonymous with cardiovascular conditioning. Since the exercise performed is within the limits of oxygen transport capability, it is also called aerobic training.

Regardless of the title, exercise is the means to fitness in the cardiac patient. An improved state of fitness is a major gain in a secondary prevention program.

Exercise Candidates and Noncandidates

Activities and exercise in the three preceding rehab phases have had prevention of deconditioning as their purpose. Now, with cardiovascular conditioning as the exercise goal, determination must be made of which patients are appropriate for exercise testing and training. Not every cardiac patient is a candidate for exercise.

Contraindications to exercise have been identified. Presence of any of the known contraindications eliminates the patient from participating in levels of exercise involved with testing and training.

Generally, the factors negating exercise can be grouped into one of three categories:
- conditions which interfere with adequate oxygen transport
- conditions which could provoke serious, possibly lethal complications
- physical or emotional conditions which reduce the likelihood of successful exercise performance. See Table 16-3 for display of specific contraindications.

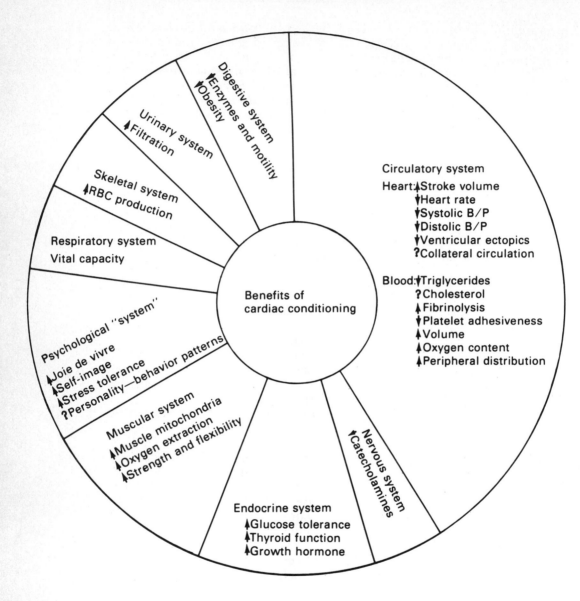

Figure 16-1. Benefits of cardiac conditioning.

Some contraindications can be labeled as "absolute." That is, exercise would never be done if existence of the condition were known or suspected, for example, dissecting aneurysm. Other contraindications might be considered "relative." Although they do represent some health deficit, the possible benefits to be gained may outweigh the risk of complication if the patient is allowed to participate cautiously in testing and training. For example, some patients with chronic atrial fibrillation gain substantial benefit from exercise training while others encounter difficulty on initial testing.

Although actual diagnosis of abnormalities is the physician's responsibility, the task of identifying and documenting contraindications is the joint responsibility of all professionals involved with Phase IV rehab care. The nursing history and cardiovascular examination are instrumental in determining presence of contraindications (see Chapter 17).

Absence of known contraindications does not mean automatic admission to the exercise test roster. Exercise testing is an elective diagnostic procedure. Exercise training is a therapeutic modality. In both circumstances, a physician's order is needed for the procedure and informed consent must be obtained from the patient.

Benefits of Exercise

Exercise is the main therapeutic thrust of Phase IV cardiac rehabilitation. Exactly how exercise contributes to cardiovascular change and fitness has been the subject of intense research. Some exercise benefits have been clearly identified and documented, while others remain theoretical or controversial.

All patients do not benefit equally from participation in exercise programs. The extent to which any patient improves is influenced by the variables at work in advance of exercise initiation. Most important to the long-term outcome are genetic endowments, previous training efforts, current level of fitness, current health status, and age.[6] Benefits gained are also affected by certain variables during training, the most significant being program fidelity and appropriate exercise prescription. Exercise training carries minimal risk and maximal effectiveness for patients who have been properly selected, appropriately tested, and professionally supervised during early training.

It is erroneous to think of cardiac exercise in terms of benefit to the heart itself. Exercise effects do not occur in such isolation, nor are cardiac changes per se necessarily the most outstanding. In fact, resulting changes in other parts of the body may make the largest contributions to improving cardiac function. Exercise benefits, therefore, may be viewed as a group of physical changes, the degree of each varying with each exercise participant. Many exercise benefits directly aid modification of other risk factors.

Although all the known physical benefits are desirable in the quest for optimal health, many authorities place primary emphasis on the psychological benefits of exercise. Obviously less measurable, but dramatically experienced by faithful exercisers, is the improved sense of well-being labeled *joie de vivre*. This natural "high" and other psychological changes accompanying it are among the reasons why exercise should be a way of life. Figure 16-1 illustrates possible exercise benefits.

Since all of the benefits shown contribute to improved physical and mental health and fitness, they are characterized as adding to the quality of life. The question of the effects of exercise on longevity, life's quantity, remains to be answered.

References

1. MOREHOUSE, L. and MILLER, A., "Circulatory Adjustments During Exercise," *Physiology of Exercise* (St. Louis, Missouri: The C. V. Mosby Company, 1971), p. 123.
2. MITCHELL, J. and BLOMQUIST, G., "Maximal Oxygen Uptake," *Physiology in Medicine*, May 1971, pp. 1018-1022.
3. DETRY, J. M., *Exercise Testing and Training in Coronary Heart Disease* (Baltimore, Maryland: Williams & Wilkins, 1973), pp. 14-15.
4. COMMITTEE on EXERCISE, *Exercise Testing and Training of Apparently Healthy Individuals: A Handbook for Physicians* (New York: American Heart Association, 1972), pp. 8-9.
5. PRESIDENT'S COUNCIL on PHYSICAL FITNESS & SPORTS, *Physical Fitness Research Digest*, No. 1, 1971.
6. FROELICHER, V., "The Hemodynamic Effects of Physical Conditioning in Healthy Young & Middle-Aged Individuals, And in Coronary Heart Disease Patients," *Exercise Testing and Exercise Training in Coronary Heart Disease* (New York: Academic Press, 1973), p. 64.

17

assessments for phase IV cardiac rehabilitation

Behaviorial Objectives

After completion of this chapter, the reader should be able to:

- state the purpose of reviewing the patient's medical and rehab history upon Phase IV entry.
- give two reasons for a nurse's cardiovascular examination prior to exercise testing and training.
- describe a practical method for conducting the pre-exercise examination.
- discuss the significance of thorough 12 lead ECG assessment prior to exercise.
- define the purpose of exercise stress testing with Phase IV cardiac rehab patients.
- select a testing method, mode, and protocol for a personal stress test (assuming availability) and discuss rationale for selection.
- describe in sequence the pretest procedure for skin prep.
- illustrate proper electrode placement for a 12 lead recording system.

Behavioral Objectives Cont'd

■ outline a procedure for routine data collection during the test.

■ name at least six abnormal responses that could occur during testing and discuss the significance of each.

■ explain how to assess ST segment changes on an exercise ECG.

Introduction

Assessment of the capabilities and needs of each patient entering a Phase IV cardiac rehab program is a nursing function. As discussed in the preceding chapter, Phase IV entry may be a progressive step in a comprehensive rehab program that began with acute admission, or it may be the patient's first encounter with organized rehabilitation efforts. In either case, results of three interrelated assessments—the nursing history, the cardiovascular examination, and the exercise stress test—lay the foundation for Phase IV cardiac rehabilitation. See Figure 17-1.

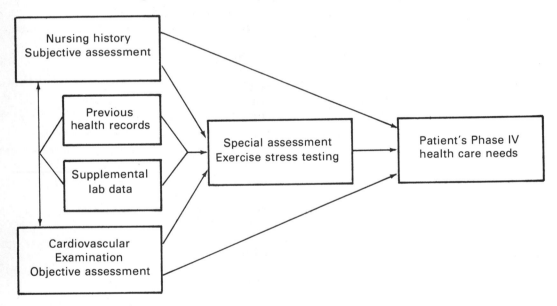

Figure 17-1.   Phase IV initial assessment structure.

The Phase IV Nursing History

Collection of a nursing history as part of an outpatient admission interview was presented in detail in Chapter 12. With a new patient entering Phase IV, the admission data collection would be gathered in the same manner. With a patient transferring from Phase III to Phase IV, the outpatient data gathered previously and built upon throughout recent weeks in Phase III are reviewed and updated as necessary in preparation for exercise testing and training.

Up to this point, exercise and activities have been of mild to moderate intensity. Exercise testing to be done here in the rehab sequence usually involves moderate- to high-intensity work in order to allow measurement of performance capability. But not every rehab patient is a candidate for exercise. For this reason, special nursing attention must be given to the review and update of the health history of every patient entering Phase IV.

Contraindications to exercise testing and training (Chapter 16) may be identified in the medical records. A history of chronic congestive heart failure, suspected aneurysm, or a fixed-rate pacemaker preclude exercise testing. Conditions which would necessitate special exercise procedures or precautions may also be found. For example, a patient with a full leg prosthesis may not be able to perform a treadmill test, but arrangements could be made for bicycle ergometer testing.

Signs and/or symptoms to anticipate during exercise testing or training may be uncovered. Patients with a history of angina, dysrhythmia, or hypertension are likely candidates for such developments during exercise performance. By knowing the patient's medications, the physician and nurse can be forewarned about certain exercise responses. Awareness of potential problems is a definite advantage for the testing physician and nurse.

Historical review of records of patients who have progressed through earlier rehab phases should provide an additional assessment "head start" for the Phase IV nurse. Nursing records will identify which objectives have been met thus far in the rehab process, which objectives remain to be accomplished, and which obstacles exist. This phase-to-phase continuum of nursing care is the ideal in cardiac rehabilitation practice.

The Cardiovascular Examination

Physical appraisal has been an important part of nursing assessment throughout rehab. Prior to Phase IV exercise, a thorough assessment of cardiovascular status is mandatory to patient safety. In addition, new or previously unidentified educational needs based on physical findings are a frequent result of the cardiovascular examination.

While physical appraisal methods and techniques are familiar to many nurse practitioners, one approach will be described here so that application to Phase IV rehab can be illustrated. A systematic approach is essential. Utilization of inspection, palpation, percussion, and auscultation will produce the best results. Skill in performing the four examination components is gained by learning the principles and practicing the techniques.

Inspection

General Appearance. As in every assessment situation, observation is a valuable tool. When the patient walks into the room, notice posture and gait. Determine the underlying problem if the patient is walking unsteadily. Does the patient have a musculoskeletal problem, a history of a CVA, or is the patient intoxicated? Some musculoskeletal problems will interfere with exercise performance or require special adaptations.

With a CVA, brain function has been compromised by a lack of blood supply. Residual effects, such as paralysis or paresthesia, may limit exercise possibilities.

Alcohol depresses the nervous system, dulling the senses. Coordination and mental alertness are drastically altered. Therefore, the exercise is risky. Use of an exercise appliance like a treadmill could result in the patient being injured from a fall. In addition, cardiac myopathy, a common complication of chronic alcoholism, may contraindicate exercise.

What is the patient's hearing potential? Does he constantly ask to have questions repeated? A hearing deficit will make clear, concise pre-exercise instructions a must. Special teaching methods may be necessary.

Does the patient wear glasses? If so, he should wear them to set accurate workloads for exercising on calibrated appliances. Safety guards should be available. Large-type teaching aids may need to be improvised for patients with severe visual handicaps.

Evaluate the patient's emotional status. Does he appear nervous and upset? An increase in sympathetic nervous activity would show a corresponding increase in heart rate and blood pressure and could postpone exercise.

Although some of the observations seem minor, variations could adversely affect the patient's exercise response.

Head and Neck. Inspection of the head and neck should include observation of color, presence of edema, xanthelasma, corneal arcus, or goiters.

To effectively evaluate skin color, a reference as to how the patient normally looks should be sought. Some description should be found in the patient's past history and physical examination reports, and questioning the patient will help confirm his normal appearance.

Cyanosis in a cardiac patient is an ominous sign. The skin, most frequently the mucous membranes of the oral cavity, the nose, lips, and earlobes exhibit a bluish discoloration. Insufficient oxygenation of arterial blood, as in pulmonary disease, or decreased circulatory performance, as in congestive heart failure, are among possible causes.

The cardiac patient who has concurrent pulmonary disease must be observed carefully during exercise for signs of insufficient oxygenation. Hypoxia is frequently indicated by early occurrence of dysrhythmia with exercise. In congestive heart failure, there is a decrease in cardiac output and, thus, a decrease in the amount of oxygen transported to the tissues. Peripheral cyanosis is a late sign of inadequacy.

It should be realized that in order for the skin to exhibit a blue color, the blood must have an absolute amount of approximately 5 Gm. unoxygenated hemoglobin. The anemic patient, who has a decreased amount of hemoglobin, will physiologically be unable to appear cyanotic.

Pallor is the descriptive term given to the skin color of the anemic patient. This lack of color is due to a decrease in the amount of circulating blood cells and/or hemoglobin. If the anemia is severe enough, it may precipitate cardiac failure, coronary insufficiency, or myocardial infarction. The anemic patient is a poor candidate for exercise because of this oxygen-carrying deficit. Cyanosis or pallor may transiently appear in a patient who is nervous or cold.

Jaundice, the result of bile pigment deposits, can be seen on the skin and mucous membranes, but is best seen on the sclera. This excess supply of bilirubin is due to any one of the many problems which can occur with the liver. The patient manifesting liver-related symptoms should be evaluated thoroughly for associated pathology before any exercise is undertaken.

Another important sign is the presence of edema. Edema of cardiac origin is usually manifested in the lower extremities, whereas edema of the face and periorbital spaces is frequently of renal origin. Therefore, in assessing the cardiac status, facial edema is not a common finding.

Xanthelasmas are small, flat, yellow lipid lesions found on the upper or lower eyelids. Such deposits are a sign of hyperlipidemia. An associated finding of the eye is corneal arcus, the presence of a gray-white ring at the junction of the sclera and cornea. This ring, which is common in the elderly (arcus senilus) and blacks is also caused by actual lipid deposits. Patients with these findings should be followed carefully with education appropriate to their diet and/or medication.

The presence of a goiter would indicate a thyroid dysfunction. The patient with hyperthyroidism may appear nervous and highly excitable. As a result of the increased metabolic rate, the heart rate and blood pressure would be elevated.

Chest and Abdomen. Inspection of the patient's chest and abdomen includes observation of respiratory movement. Breathing patterns should be noted and abnormal findings thoroughly investigated. (See Chapter 7 for a review of respiratory assessments.)

Inspection may reveal an increased anterior-posterior chest diameter indicative of chronic obstructive pulmonary disease. This patient should be watched closely for signs of hypoxia with exercise.

Xanthomas, like xanthelasmas, are small, yellow, lipid lesions. Xanthomas are found on any part of the body. Descriptive names have been given to the xanthomas depending on their type or the area of the body on which they appear. Eruptive xanthomas are found in clusters resembling a rash and may be located on the chest, abdomen, and back. Xanthomas are also a sign of hyperlipidemia.

Extremities. Edema of cardiac origin is first seen in the lower extremities. It is caused by increased venous pressure which interrupts return of fluid to the heart. As a result, the fluid escapes into the interstitial spaces. Edema may be pitting and can be graded according to severity—a + 4 (very deep) to a trace (barely an imprint). The gradation of edema is extremely subjective and is best utilized when a comparison is based upon the established norm in a given hospital. Chronic edema, seen in patients with chronic right heart failure, will feel woody.

If the edema is unilateral, the patient should be evaluated for the presence of varicosities, thrombophlebitis, or an occlusion of an artery. Patients with severe varicosities may develop leg fatigue early in exercise.

To evaluate for the presence of thrombophlebitis or clotting of the deep veins, dorsiflex the foot. If the patient complains of calf pain, it is a positive Homans' sign indicative of thrombophlebitis.

An occlusion of an artery would produce cyanosis and edema of the affected limb. Both peripheral occlusion and thrombophlebitis are obvious contraindications to exercise. The risk of dislodging the thrombus and causing a pulmonary embolus is great.

Hair distribution on the toes and lowers legs and color and thickness of toenails should be evaluated. Arterial insufficiency (arteriosclerosis) may cause hair on the lower extremities to fall out and toenails to become thick and yellowed.

As mentioned previously, xanthomas may occur on the extremities. One common area is on the Achilles tendon. On first glance, patients with xanthomas may appear to have thick ankles.

On the upper extremities, clubbing is one of the most prominent, but late, signs. An abnormally high blood flow caused by chronic tissue hypoxia causes accelerated tissue growth at the ends of the fingers. This extra tissue causes the fingers to look like clubs. Tissue hypoxia of this type is seen in chronic obstructive pulmonary disease and certain types of congenital heart disease.[1]

Palpation

The second step of the physical appraisal process is very effective if done along with inspection of the patient. As the nurse is palpating various areas of the body, she can observe closely for color, edema, and so on.

Pulses. To assure that an adequate blood supply is being pumped throughout the body, pulses should be palpated (see Table 17-1). While checking the pulse, one extremity should be compared to its symmetrical opposite. The carotid pulses should be palpated one at a time.

Table 17-1
Pre-exercise Pulse Checks

Location	Rationale
Carotid	Inadequate cerebral perfusion may result in the exercising patient becoming disoriented, syncopal, or in extreme cases, experiencing a CVA.
Radial	Inadequate perfusion to a hand or arm may result in pain, difficult to distinguish from referred angina.

Lower extremity pulses
  Popliteal
  Posterior tibial
  Dorsalis pedis
	Inadequate perfusion to the lower extremities may result in leg fatigue, or in more severe cases, claudication.

The pulse should be evaluated for presence, rate, rhythm, and amplitude. A diminished pulse in one extremity could indicate a unilateral arterial occlusion. A distortion of rhythm or rate would necessitate a more thorough evaluation for dysrhythmia such as ectopics or tachydysrhythmias. Depending on the nature of the rhythm abnormality, exercise may be contraindicated. The forcefulness of cardiac output is evaluated by the amplitude of the pulse. Excitement, heat, and exercise may all cause an increase in stroke volume.

Many types of pulses have been identified, usually in association with specific disease entities (see Table 17-2).

Chest. While palpating the chest area, be alert for the presence of vibrations over the four major valve areas (see Figure 17-2). These vibrations are called thrills and are associated with loud murmurs. Thrills are usually felt in cases of valvular stenosis rather than regurgitation.

The PMI, or point of maximal intensity, is normally palpated about the fifth intercostal space at the midclavicular line. Displacement may be seen in patients with left ventricular hypertrophy, ascites, or a tumor. These problems are also detectable by·x-ray examination of the chest.

Abdomen. Increased aortic pulsations in the abdominal region could be indicative of an abdominal aortic aneurysm. Because of the increased force of contraction and pressure against the wall of the aorta, exercise could cause the aneurysm to rupture.

Percussion

Percussion is not as useful as other assessment methods for the nurse evaluating an outpatient entering an exercise program. The tapping procedure can be used to outline the size of organs, but tends to be very subjective. Most of the data obtained by percussion can be determined through the use of more reliable tools such as x-ray studies.

Auscultation

Listening to sounds being emitted through the chest wall is a skill that requires continual practice. A good stethoscope is a must for good auscultation. It should have a bell to hear low-pitched sounds, a diaphragm to detect high-pitched sounds, and be no longer than 60 cm. or 24 inches.

Blood Pressure. Blood pressure measurements are frequently taken for granted by experienced nurses. A review of technique is helpful from time to time. Proper technique will eliminate false high or false low readings (see Table 17-3).

Comparison of blood pressures in both arms is essential. A difference of 10 mm. Hg or more between arms would warrant closer observation. Provided proper technique is being used, an arterial compression or obstruction would be suspected with an extreme deviation. A dissecting aortic aneurysm can cause a variation in the readings between arms.

Repeated blood pressure readings for comparison should be taken in the patient with suspected hypertension. Anxiety is one of the most frequent causes of inconsistent high blood pressure readings.

Table 17-2
Pulse Abnormalities by Palpation

Name	Characteristics	Associations
Pulsus magnus (also called Corrigan's pulse or water-hammer pulse)	Forceful pulse Rises and falls rapidly Associated with wide pulse pressure	Aortic insufficiency Severe anemia Systolic hypertension Hyperthyroidism
Pulsus parvus	Slow small pulse Rises and falls slowly Associated with narrow pulse pressure	Aortic stenosis Mitral stenosis Hypotension Left Ventricular failure (Due to increased stroke volume)
Pulsus paradoxus or paradoxical pulse	Decreased pulse amplitude with inspiration Abnormal finding if heard during relaxed respirations Best determined while auscultating blood pressure	Severe COPD Constrictive pericarditis
Pulsus bigeminus or bigeminal pulse	Irregular rhythm Normal beat alternating with premature beats Can be confused with pulsus alternans	Myocardial irritability producing dysrhythmias
Pulsus alternans or alternating pulse	Regular rhythm Every other beat is weak Best determined while auscultating the blood pressure	Left ventricular failure Severe hypertension

Table 17-3
Technical Problems in Auscultating Blood Pressure

Cause	Cure
False High Blood Pressure Readings	
1. Initial inflation too slow	1. Inflate rapidly
2. Inflated too high	2. Inflate 20-30 mm. Hg above the point at which the radial pulse disappears
3. Use of regular-sized cuff on obese arm	3. Use large cuff on obese arm
4. Patient holding arm out stiffly (isometric)	4. Have arm relaxed and supported
False Low Blood Pressure Readings	
Use of regular-sized cuff on thin arm	Use a small cuff on thin arm
Inability to Hear Blood Pressure	
Repeated cuff inflation causes venous engorgement	Allow relaxation time between repeat attempts

Heart Sounds. The heart should be auscultated for the presence of gallops, murmurs, and rubs. The presence of any one of these abnormalities should prompt a request for thorough medical investigation before the initiation of exercise.

Auscultation of heart sounds should be performed systematically, taking care to listen closely to the specific valvular areas as seen in Figure 17-2. The auscultation should be done by moving the stethoscope slowly from one area to the next, alternating bell and diaphragm, also pausing to listen between areas. Following a "Z" pattern is helpful.

To review, the first heart sound (S_1) is caused by the closure of the mitral and tricuspid valves. The second heart sound (S_2) is caused by the closure of the aortic and pulmonic valves. The S_1 or S_2 can sound split. This is normal in many people and is due to the fact that the valves do not close exactly together. When

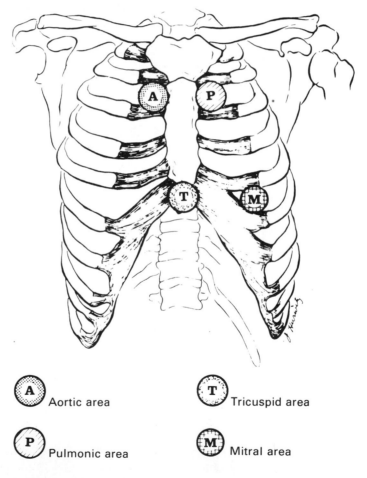

Figure 17-2.   Chest areas for auscultation of heart sounds.

there is a wide split in the sound, the nurse must determine if the sound is a split heart sound or a gallop rhythm. For example, a split S_2 is seen in pulmonic stenosis and right bundle-branch block.

In patients with a noncompliant left ventricle, a third heart sound (S_3) may develop. This is most often seen in heart failure and is also called a ventricular gallop. A physiological third heart sound may be heard in young adults and children, but is not a normal finding in a cardiac patient.

A fourth heart sound (S_4) is heard prior to S_1 and is called an artrial gallop. The artrial sound is made prominent by forceful atrial contraction against a ventricle which has developed increased resistance to filling. It is not necessarily associated with noncompliance of the left ventricle as seen in congestive heart failure.

An S_4 may be heard in patients who have coronary artery disease, hypertensive cardiovascular disease, or aortic stenosis. An electrical problem which causes a delay in conduction from the atria to the ventricles would also cause vibration of blood in the atria and, thus, an S_4. The presence of an S_4 does not necessarily contraindicate exercise.

Murmurs are vibrations caused by turbulent blood flow through a stenosed or insufficient valve. They are also caused by the vibration of blood which has lost its viscosity as seen in anemia. Any type of valve problem will eventually affect the cardiac output. This compromised output may cause a multitude of problems during exercise.

If a murmur is heard, it should be identified as to quality, pitch, timing, grade, location, and radiation. The following descriptive detail will help determine the underlying problem:

- The quality of the murmur indicates if it is loud, harsh, rumbling, and so on.
- The pitch, high or low, is best determined by using both the bell and diaphragm of the stethoscope.
- Timing of the murmur is the determination if it is heard in systole or diastole. For a diagramatic review, see Figure 17-3.
- Grading murmurs is a very subjective procedure. They are usually classified Grade I (barely audible) to Grade VI (booming). Grades I, II, and sometimes Grade III are many times functional or nonpathological murmurs.
- Location and radiation will determine where on the chest the murmur is heard best.

The murmur of mitral insufficiency is systolic in time and is heard best at the apex or mitral valve area. A common cause of this murmur in cardiac patients is papillary muscle dysfunction. It's seriousness should be evaluated with the rest of the clinical findings to determine if exercise is contraindicated.

The murmur of mitral stenosis is diastolic in time and is also heard best at the apex. Mitral stenosis may initiate atrial fibrillation during an exercise stress test.[2]

Aortic stenosis will greatly alter the cardiac output and may constitute canceling exercise, especially an exercise stress test. The murmur of aortic stenosis is systolic in time and heard best in the second right intercostal space.

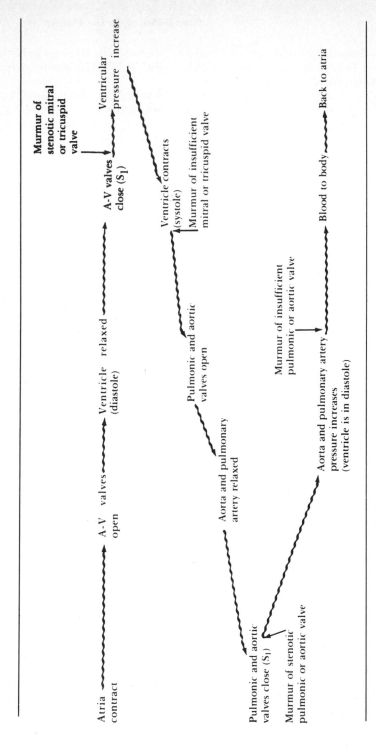

Figure 17-3. Review of cardiac cycle and relationship of murmurs. ($\sim\!\!\!\!\sim\!\!\!\!\blacktriangleright$ blood flow)

The murmur of aortic insufficiency is diastolic in time and is heard at the second right interspace. The presence of this murmur does not always contra-indicate stress testing.

When auscultating the heart, a friction rub caused by inflammation of the pericardial sac may be heard throughout the cardiac cycle. The underlying acute inflammatory process is a contraindication to exercise.

Lung Sounds. The presence of râles or rhonchi on auscultation of the lungs could be a sign of any pulmonary problem from pulmonary edema to pneumonia. The cause of abnormal lung sounds is usually diagnosed by x-ray examination.

While auscultating the lungs, a pleural friction rub may be heard. This is caused by inflammation of the pleura. To differentiate the two types of rubs, have the patient hold his breath. If the rub is still heard, it is pericardial not pleural (see Chapter 7 for a review of breath sounds).

Tests and Procedures

Various other tools should also be used to evaluate the patient entering Phase IV rehab. These comprise a fifth category of physical appraisal which includes vital signs, height and weight, vital capacity, 12 lead ECG, x-ray exami-nation of the chest, and blood studies.

Vital Signs. Temperature is an important factor in overall assessment of the patient. A fever could be a sign of almost any type of illness, so an elevated temperature should prompt further investigation as to the cause. During exercise, metabolism increases, thus increasing body temperature. Patients with undetected low-grade fevers may develop dizziness, fainting, or other symptoms of heat exhaustion.

The *apical rate* should be taken while auscultating the chest, noting rate and rhythm.

The *respiratory rate* should also be counted. Observe the patient's breathing for type and quality. Abnormal patterns should be investigated.

Height and Weight. Height and weight are often overlooked as more dramatic information is sought. In the cardiac patient, a weight gain could indicate fluid accumulation, such as that seen in heart failure. A more common cause of weight gain is overeating. An obese patient would have special teaching needs. Both height and weight should be measured. When asked, patients tend to understate weight and overstate height.

Pulmonary Function Tests. Vital capacity is a measurement of how much air is forceably exhaled after a full inspiration. It is frequently performed prior to exercise testing as a screening test for pulmonary dysfunction. A below average reading could indicate a restrictive problem, such as a tumor pressing on the lung inhibiting full expansion.

A one-second forced expiratory volume (FEV_1) and a three-second forced expiratory volume (FEV_3) are measurements of the amount of air the patient can blow out in one and three seconds. These values are compared to the patient's vital capacity. If these values fall below the norm, it could indicate an obstructive lung problem, such as emphysema.

The 12 Lead ECG. The Phase IV rehab nurse must have a working knowledge of what constitutes a normal and abnormal ECG.

If the patient is to undergo an exercise stress test, a standard 12 lead ECG *must* be done prior to the test. The patient's ECG should be evaluated for problems that would either contraindicate exercise or would necessitate close observation throughout the exercise. Table 17-4 presents a summary of major ECG abnormalities and their usefulness in pre-exercise assessment.

Table 17-4
Pre-exercise Assessment: The Standard 12 Lead ECG

ECG Abnormality	Pre-exercise Significance
ST segment elevation	Absolute contraindications
Acute MI; if "silent" may not have been identified from history	
Pericarditis	
2nd- or 3rd-degree A-V block	Contraindications, due to cardiac output limitations
Fixed rate pacemakers	
Accelerated conduction	Caution; patients have a tendency toward spontaneous tachydysrhythmia
Lown-Ganong-Levine	
Wolf-Parkinson-White	
Left bundle-branch block	Caution; left bundle-branch block may be related to diminished left ventricular function; pattern interferes with ischemic ST segment manifestations
Ventricular ectopics	
Occasional, unifocal	Proceed; carefully observe ectopic occurrence
Frequent, multifocal, short coupling intervals, runs	Contraindications
Left ventricular hypertrophy	Caution; may limit cardiac output
Atrial fibrillation flutter	Caution; ventricular response and cardiac output unpredictable
Electrolyte abnormalities	Contraindications; either potassium extreme can be life-threatening
Hypokalemia	
Hyperkalemia	

The main point to remember when evaluating pre-exercise ECGs is to look for changes on the ECG that weren't on previous tracings. If changes are seen, determine what they are and what could cause them. Then discuss with the physician if the patient is a safe candidate for exercise.

Lab Studies. Lab studies such as CBC, x-ray examination of the cholesterol triglyceride, and electrolytes should be done prior to an exercise stress test. These are utilized as screening devices just as the ECG.

    1. The CBC results would indicate if the patient is anemic. The severity of the anemia would determine if the exercise should be undertaken.

2. The x-ray examination of the chest will show abnormalities of structure, such as cardiac enlargement, aneurysm, and the like. The lungs would also show fluid or consolidation.
3. Cholesterol and triglyceride levels should be measured to determine what type of dietary counseling is needed, if any.
4. Electrolyte levels will show if any supplements or changes in treatment are warranted prior to exercise, the potassium level being the most important consideration.

Documentation

Once the physical appraisal is completed, documentation should be undertaken. Any method as long as it is done in a logical manner will suffice. Keep comments clear and concise.

Documentation should include all facets of the appraisal (see Table 17-5 for a sample format). Problems identified as a result of this assessment should be summarized at the conclusion of the examination report.

The Exercise Stress Test

Definition and Purpose

Cardiac performance is altered by any increased physical or psychological activity. The body demands cardiac compensation regardless of the source of "stress." For example, rushing to catch the morning commuter train, getting angry with a boss, or walking on a treadmill in a diagnostic laboratory may summon similar responses. Knowing in advance if a given cardiac patient is capable of generating the responses needed for such situations is a function of exercise stress testing.

By definition, exercise stress testing is "the observation and recording of an individual's responses during a measured exercise challenge in order to determine his capacity to adapt to physical stress."[3] Information obtained is useful in planning both medical and nursing care in cardiac rehabilitation. Test results will aid the nurse in selecting an appropriate exercise program for the patient, in answering questions regarding occupations or activities of daily living, and in arranging assistance and motivation for necessary changes in lifestyle.

Exercise stress testing may also be called work evaluation, exercise tolerance testing, or functional capacity determination. Regardless of the label applied, the purpose of such testing with a postacute cardiac patient is the same—measurement of the safe extent of cardiac adaptability. Testing of this nature is usually first performed six to twelve weeks following acute cardiac event.

Professional Responsibilities

Exercise tests may be performed in a hospital's diagnostic cardiovascular lab, a doctor's office, a cardiac rehab unit, or in other ambulatory care settings. According to the American Heart Association:

Table 17-5
Assessment Guide for Nurse's Cardiovascular Examination

I. Inspection

A. General appearance

1. Posture and gait
2. Hearing
3. Glasses
4. Mental status

B. Head and neck

1. Color
2. Edema
3. Xanthelasmas
4. Corneal arcus
5. Goiter

C. Chest and abdomen
1. Movement
2. A-P diameter
3. Xanthomas

D. Extremities

1. Edema
3. Homans' sign
4. Hair distribution and toenails
5. Xanthomas
6. Clubbing

II. Palpation

A. Pulses (List each site separately)

1. Quality
2. Rate
3. Rhythm
4. Amplitude

B. Chest

1. Thrills
2. PMI

C. Abdomen

Pulsations

III. Percussion

Not applicable for purposes of this examination

IV. Auscultation

A. Blood pressure (both arms)
B. Heart sounds
C. Lung sounds

V. Special tests and procedures
A. Vital signs
B. Height
C. Weight
D. Vital capacity*
E. 12 lead ECG
F. X-ray examination of the chest*
G. Blood studies*

* Obtain results from other labs.

Responsibility for prescribing, supervising, interpreting, reporting and recommending (exercise) testing and training belongs to the physician. Direct physician supervision of testing and training sessions, while desirable, is not always necessary *provided* the health care personnel directing the sessions are trained to the satisfaction of the responsible physician in cardiopulmonary resuscitation and emergency cardiac care according to the standards set by the American Heart Association and the Committee on Emergency Medical Services of the National Academy of Sciences, National Research Council, Division of Medical Sciences. Such individuals should have the capability and authorization to perform cardiopulmonary resuscitation, including electrical defibrillation. Such authorization may require changes in some state laws.[4]

Since nurses practicing in cardiovascular care areas are usually trained and experienced in basic cardiopulmonary resuscitation, defibrillation, and advanced life support techniques, they are frequently sought out to organize and operate exercise-testing units. Although a nurse may be responsible for managing a testing lab, it is a medicolegal policy of most institutions that a physician conduct exercise testing on known cardiac patients.

Ideally, the same nurse who will be working with the patient throughout Phase IV of his rehab program should be involved with each of the major assessments—the nursing history, the cardiovascular examination, and the exercise stress test. If it is not possible for the rehab nurse to actually participate in the testing procedure, she should at least (where physically possible) observe the patient's test performance. Firsthand observation may result in a nursing care insight not likely to be transmitted through routine test reports.

Risks and Precautions

Rare Events. Exercise stress testing is not risk free. Rare episodes of acute cardiac events, such as myocardial infarction, and even more rarely, death, have been documented. In the most extensive study, Rochmis and Blackburn surveyed 170,000 tests and found:

> A combined complication rate of the deaths and nonfatal events requiring hospitalization within one week (of the exercise stress test) is about 66 per 170,000 or about 4 per 10,000 (0.04%). Sixteen documented deaths were attributed to the exercise, giving a death rate of about 1 per 10,000 tests (0.01%). Approximately 40 subjects were reported to have been hospitalized in the immediate period following an exercise test for events which proved to be nonfatal, a rate of 2.4 per 10,000 tests (0.02%).[5]

In comparison, mortality is much less than that for coronary arteriography.[6]

To help assure optimal safety, nurses involved with exercise testing, either as staff members of a testing facility or as rehab nurses following specific patients, should assume coresponsibility with the testing physician in two areas of pretest preparation. First, the existence of contraindications to exercise performance must be ruled out (see Chapter 16). The elimination of high-risk patients is the major purpose of nursing history and cardiovascular examination upon Phase IV entry. Second, emergency preparation is essential in any health care setting routinely visited by cardiac patients, including testing facilities (see discussion of emergency preparation in Chapter 14, Unit III).

General Precautions. In addition to morbidity and mortality, consideration should also be given to general discomfort or anxiety as a "risk" associated with exercise testing. If a patient has any unpleasant experience associated with the testing procedure, his attitude about exercise could be negatively influenced. Prevention of most undesirable responses can be effected by good nursing care.

Advance Instructions. Prior to his test appointment, perhaps in conjunction with his admission interview or by follow-up phone conversation, the patient needs to be instructed as to the do's and don'ts of exercise testing.

1. Exercise should not be performed with a full stomach since digestion creates a conflicting demand with exercise for oxygen; avoid eating for two to four hours before the test (if the test is to be done in early morning, fasting should be from the night before).

2. Exercise should not be performed within two to four hours of cigarette smoking; nicotine increases heart rate, and the carbon monoxide in cigarette smoke can interfere with oxygen transport because of the affinity of hemoglobin for carbon monoxide; ideally, this brief cessation would be step 1 of a total smoking withdrawal program.

3. Exercise should not be performed within two to four hours of ingestion of any caffeinated beverage, such as coffee, tea, or cola, since caffeine increases heart rate.

4. Appropriate exercise clothing should be suggested: Men should wear shorts or loose-fitting pants. Women should wear shorts or loose-fitting pants, a short-line cotton bra, a short-sleeved front-buttoned shirt, and socks or knee-hi's (no pantyhose). Both should wear sneakers or other flat walking or running shoes.

In addition, patients should be advised of the approximate length of time they will be in the testing lab so that time-related stress is eliminated.

Exercise Environment. The exercise environment should be checked prior to test performance; the ideal exercise environment is 20° to 21°C (68° to 72°F) with a humidity of less than 50 percent.[7] Higher temperatures inhibit convective heat loss. Higher humidity suppresses evaporation of perspiration.

Medications. The patient should be questioned about all medications he's been taking. The possibility of drug-influenced responses or side effects must be identified in advance (see Chapter 19). It is not usually necessary to discontinue medications when a test is being done to determine functional capacity. In fact, if the patient is to participate in the exercise-training program while on medication, he *should* be tested on those medications.[8]

Informed Consent. As with any diagnostic procedure, the patient has the right to be informed about the test procedure he is about to undergo and the possible risks and complications involved. Responsibility for imparting information concerning potential hazards and then obtaining the patient's permission to take related risks belongs to the physician. The nurse is the usual witness to the patient's signature on the informed consent record.

Pretest Instructions. Immediately preceding test performance, specific instructions should be given to the patient to reduce the possibility of injury or side effects.

1. The patient should be acclimated to the testing apparatus; he should be shown how to mount and dismount the treadmill (or other device); a brief practice walk will help reduce machine anxiety.

2. The patient should be instructed to breathe normally during the test, but to expect his breathing rate to increase; both Valsalva maneuvers and hyperventilation are undesirable; the patient should be cautioned not to hold his breath (a natural inclination at high levels of work on the bicycle ergometer) and not to breathe too shallowly.

3. The patient should be instructed to walk on a treadmill without holding onto the safety rails, if possible; if balance becomes a problem, a light touch of a finger or two will help maintain position; gripping the bar is an isometric contraction and is to be avoided.

4. The patient should be informed of the expected sequence of the test (warm-up, progressive test performance, and recovery).

5. The patient should be informed that he has a right to request that the test be discontinued at any point if he so desires.

6. The patient should be told to expect to work hard and "be sweaty."

7. The patient should be told to advise the nurse or doctor immediately if he experiences any discomfort.

8. After the test, if shower facilities are available, the patient should be instructed to take a tepid shower, not a hot one. Hot water will rapidly cause vasodilatation in the skin, and fainting and injury could result from the sudden circulation shift.

Methods, Modes, and Protocols

A variety of approaches to exercise stress testing is currently in use. Nurses practicing in cardiac care areas may be familiar with the more common types of tests utilized. As a specialist, the nurse in the exercise-testing lab must know the rationale for the methods preferred by her institution, have total familiarity with the equipment chosen, be well-versed in the protocols preferred by the testing physicians, and most important, realize the importance and appropriateness of testing choices to the patient as an individual.

Methods. Testing methods can be subdivided into several alternative approaches.

1. An exercise stress test may be maximal or submaximal.

    In physiological terms, a maximal test exercises an individual to a level of intensity beyond which further increase in the magnitude of work will not be accompanied by increased oxygen uptake; the individual has attained his maximal oxygen uptake. A maximal test defines the true state of cardiovascular fitness of an individual whether he is an athlete, a sedentary normal adult, or a cardiac patient.[9]

    Determination of the point at which this maximal transport occurs can be directly measured by blood sampling and/or pulmonary testing during exercise. Since such additional procedures are frequently cumbersome for the staff and anxiety-provoking to the patient, extrapolation of oxygen transport information is often done from tables and formulas based on previously measured "norms."

    Practically speaking, heart rate serves as a useful indicator of when a maximal test has been accomplished. When no further increase in heart rate results from increased work, it can be assumed that a maximal oxygen transport level has been reached.

Prior to test initiation, there is no way of knowing what an individual's maximal heart rate will be. Although many studies have generated "predicted" maximal heart rates based on study populations, heart rate values given are not consistent from study to study and, therefore, applying predictions to individuals is of limited usefulness.

Sheffield and his coworkers studied groups of men in an attempt to define maximal heart rates and found that age and physical condition were the two factors having the biggest influence on maximal heart rate attained during exercise stress.[10] Trends at least can be anticipated. Older individuals will have lower maximal heart rates; more physically fit individuals will have lower maximal heart rates than the sedentary adult.

A submaximal test is one in which a test is terminated at a pre-determined heart rate, usually 85 percent of the maximum age-predicted heart rate.[11] Use of the arbitrary submaximal test limit is considered appropriate for some functional evaluations, since an 85 percent (of age-predicted maximum) achievement is sufficient enough to provide information needed to determine exercise prescriptions (see Table 17-6).

Contrary to what might be expected, submaximal testing does not provide a lower risk to the patient than maximal testing. The survey of Rochmis and Blackburn could not identify a relationship between mortality and the type of test (submaximal or maximal).[12]

Currently, the type of test being done most often with known cardiac patients has come to be called functional capacity or symptom-limited testing. The test progresses until the patient is exhausted or an abnormal sign, symptom, or ECG change occurs. The point at which the abnormality occurs may or may not coincide with maximal heart rate, although truly representing the patient's maximal performance ability.

Table 17-6
Averages of Maximal Heart Rates Published by
Ten American and European Investigators

Ages by Decades	20-29	30-39	40-49	50-59	60-69
MHR	190	182	179	171	164

Adapted from Exercise and Stress Testing Workshop Report, "Exercise, Proceedings of the National Workshop on Exercise." *The Journal of the South Carolina Medical Association,* December 1969, Supplement, p. 75.

2. An exercise stress test may be single-stage or multistage.

A single-stage test is one in which the same arbitrary level of work is performed throughout the duration of the test. The Master 2 Step is a classic example. The major advantage of a single-stage test is the simplicity of both performance and equipment.

A multistage test is one in which the levels of work start low and increase progressively at regular intervals until a test goal is reached or symptoms limit further performance. Multistage testing is preferred by most testing labs. The American Heart Association Committee on Exercise states that multistage exercise testing accompanied by continuous ECG monitoring and periodic blood pressure determination is the most informative type of testing.[13]

3. An exercise stress test may be intermittent or continuous.

In an intermittent exercise test, the patient performs a specific work level and then is allowed a period of recovery before the next work level is performed. In a continuous test, the level of work is gradually increased (multistage) without interruption until the test goal is reached or symptoms limit further performance.

Continuous tests seem to be performed more often than intermittent tests probably due to the fact that total test time is obviously less. However, supporters of intermittent testing have strong points in their favor. Hellerstein states: "The continuous method of testing should not be used, because most (exercise) training (programs) is not continuous but intermittent . . . And, in the world where people work, they don't work continuously, but intermittently".[14]

Regardless of the method preferred, exercise stress testing as done with cardiac patients consists of dynamic, rhythmic, isotonic activity.

Modes. The classic forerunner of the growing sophistication associated with exercise testing today was the Master 2 Step test. Specifications for the 2 step apparatus required each step to be 22.5 cm. or 9 inches high and 25 cm. or 10 inches deep. The apparatus was solidly constructed, simple to use, and inexpensive, but it lacked capability for measuring work being done.

An erg is a unit of work. An ergometer is an apparatus for measuring work. Calibrated stationary bicycles and treadmills are the most commonly used ergometers in exercise-tesing facilities.

Bicycle Ergometer. There is a wide selection of bicycle ergometers on the current health market. Both mechanical and electromechanical bicycle ergometers are used in exercise labs.

The biggest advantage of testing with a bicycle ergometer is that the resulting ECG is generally artifact free. The ECG clarity is due to modified limb lead placements on the torso with electrodes and lead wires virtually undisturbed by pedaling action. Other advantages include low cost, little space requirement, and low maintenance.

The biggest disadvantage of the bicycle ergometer is that the muscles necessary for bicycling are generally not well developed in the U. S. population and, therefore, performance rarely reaches maximal levels.[15] Protocols for bicycle ergometer testing generally follow increments of 150 kilogram meters each stage.

Treadmill. The treadmill is the preferred modality for exercise testing in this country. According to Ellestad, the treadmill applies a more physiological workload than the bicycle ergometer. Subjects are much more likely to reach their aerobic capacity or their peak predicted heart rate on the treadmill, especially if they are not athletic in nature.[16]

The biggest disadvantage of treadmill testing is that the walking-running motion introduces ECG artifact and makes blood pressure measurement difficult. Treadmill variables (speed and grade) have been designed into a number of test protocols. An appropriate test can be selected to fit each patient. Some of the common treadmill protocols are listed in Table 17-7.

Test Technique

During exercise stress testing, the nurse and the physician are responsible for observing and evaluating patient responses. To assure that information gathered from the test is accurate and meaningful, strict attention must be given to patient preparation prior to testing and to equipment operation during testing.

Choices of monitoring-recording systems to be used in the testing lab are increasing daily. The optimal exercise-testing system is the one that provides the information desired by the lab, that the staff is capable of handling, and that the budget allows. Certain equipment functions are considered essential to testing, others are totally elective (see Table 17-8).

Single-lead bipolar systems, multilead systems (from 3 to 15 leads in various combinations), and the standard 12 lead system are all in use for exercise testing. Controversy continues as to which bipolar lead is most appropriate for testing. Both CM5 and CC5 have been well supported (see discussion of bipolar applications, Chapter 14).[17-18]

Use of the familiar 12 lead ECG system for testing requires some modification. It is neither practical nor safe to apply limb leads in their usual wrist/ankle positions on a patient about to exercise. Therefore, modified limb lead placements as recommended by Mason and Likar are required[19] (see Figure 17-4).

By far, the biggest technical problem with exercise testing is motion artifact. Muscle interference on an exercise ECG can render a test useless. Although some computerized systems have managed to overcome the motion problem, most testing facilities continue to rely on meticulous skin prep and electrode placement to minimize artifact. Table 17-9 outlines a pretest prep sequence.

In addition to determining ECG techniques for testing, a method of obtaining pressure must also be selected. Most labs use standard antecubital blood pressure measurements, although some use an anesthesia-type stethoscope with the diaphragm strapped on the arm over the brachial artery.

Table 17-7
Common Protocols for Exercise Stress Testing on Treadmills

Title	Initial Level	Progressive Levels	Stage Duration
Balke I	3 mph 0%	Maintain 3 mph Progress 2.5% each stage	2 Min.
Balke II	3.4 mph 2%	Maintain 3.4 mph Progress 2% each stage	2. Min.
Bruce	1.7 mph 10%	2.5 mph/3.4 mph/4.2 mph/5.0 mph/5.5 mph/6.0 mph 12% 14% 16% 18% 20% 22%	3 Min.
Ellestad	1.7 mph 10%	3 mph/4 mph/5 mph/6 mph 10% 10% 15% 15%	3′ /2′ /2′ /3′ /3′ /2′
Fletcher and Cantwell	2 mph 0%	Maintain 2 mph Progress 2.5% each stage	2-1/2 Min.
Katus	1.0 mph 10%	Progress 0.5 mph each stage Maintain 10%	3 min.
Naughton	2.0 mph 0%	Maintain 2 mph 3.5% / progress 3.5% each stage	2 Min.
Sheffield and Reeves	1.7 mph 0%	1.7 mph/1.7 mph/2.5 mph/3.4 mph/4.2 mph/5 mph/5.5 mph 5% 10% 12% 14% 16% 18% 20%	3. Min.

Adapted from Bruce, R. A., et al., "Maximal Oxygen Intake and Nomographic Assessment of Functional Aerobic Impairment in Cardiovascular Disease," *American Heart Journal*, Vol. 85, No. 4, April 1973, p. 549; Ellestad, M. H., *Stress Testing, Principles and Practice* (Philadelphia: F. A. Davis Company, 1975), p. 69; Fletcher, G. and Cantwell, J., *Exercise in the Management of Coronary Heart Disease* (Springfield, Illinois: Charles C Thomas, 1971), p. 16; Kattus, A. A., "Exercise Electrocardiography: Recognition of the Ischemic Response, False Positive & Negative Patterns," *American Journal of Cardiology*, May 20, 1974, p. 722; Naughton, J. P., "The Contribution of Regular Physical Activity to the Ambulatory Care of Cardiac Patients," *Postgraduate Medicine*, April 1975, p. 53; and Sheffield, T., "The Whys and Hows of Stress Testing," *Medical Opinion*, Vol. 4, No. 6, June 1975, p. 38.

Table 17-8
Component Considerations for Exercise-Testing Systems

Minimal Functions	Intermediate Capabilities	Computerized "Extras"
Single-lead system (hardwire or telemetry)	Multilead system (hardwire or telemetry)	ECG programmer Automatically records ECG at specified times; may also indicate selected ECG values on digital display, e.g., heart rate, ST segment depression
Oscilloscope display ("bouncing ball" or nonfade)	Multichannel nonfade oscilloscope	
Strip recorder*	Multichannel ECG recorder* with real time and delay record capability	Sequence programmer
Stop watch	Digital elapsed timer	Automatically advances exercise device to preprogrammed levels at specified times
	Digital heart rate meter	

*Any ECG recorder used for exercise stress testing must meet American Heart Association diagnostic frequency standards. (.05 - 100Hz)

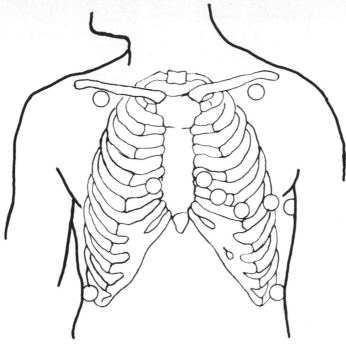

Figure 17-4. Modified 12 lead system for exercise testing.

Table 17-9
Skin Prep and Electrode Placement

1. Inform the patient of the purpose of the skin preparation.

2. Select appropriate electrode sites: electrodes must be positioned where they can be stabilized both to assure adhesiveness and to reduce motion; flat areas away from major muscles and fat pads are generally best.

3. Shave electrode sites of visible hair.

4. Cleanse the skin with acetone or alcohol to remove surface oil.

5. Rub the skin with rough gauze or fine sandpaper to remove the horny layer of epidermis: sites should be erythematous.

6. Attach electrodes firmly to the skin: either disposable or reusable electrodes may be used. Disposables have the advantage of being fast and neat, which in a busy lab is well worth the few cents more in costs. Electrodes used in other areas of the hospital, like CCU, will not necessarily function well for testing; the adhesive is frequently too weak to endure the profuse perspiration and the gel saline content may be insufficient to rapidly reduce skin resistance.

7. Secure lead wires to electrodes: it may be necessary to loop wires and secure with adhesive tape to take up slack or to reduce tugging on the electrode; adhesive should be used selectively since the added surface contact could introduce motion artifact.

8. Stabilize all lead wires and cable connectors: some systems provide special holders or belts for securing wiring. Heavy tape, an elastic bandage, or an abdominal binder can be used effectively to imobilize the system.

The latter approach can save time in taking blood pressures during testing. Few labs are using automatic blood pressure devices. Cost is a factor, but more important, reliability is less than expected during high-level exercise. Sensors are easily confused by motion artifact.

Responses During Exercise Stress Testing

Response exhibited during exercise stress provide vital information to total health assessment of the patient. Such information is needed in planning both medical and nursing care. Therefore, both physician and nurse should observe the patient's test performance.

Frequently, the nurse assumes the role of data collector operating the monitoring equipment and documenting responses. Before the testing protocol is started, reference information must be gathered. The pretest heart rate and blood pressure are measured and two ECGs recorded from electrodes in modified limb positions (on the torso). The first is recorded with the patient lying down for comparison with previous standard ECGs (amplitude may be lower in limb leads with modified placement) and postexercise supine ECGs. The second is measured with the patient in an upright position as he will be throughout the test when his ECG is recorded.

The selected test protocol is started after warm-up to allow time for the cardiovascular system to gradually adapt to exercise demands. Various procedures of collecting routine in-progress test data have been developed. Table 17-10 presents a sample approach.

In addition to the routine notations, other responses are observed throughout testing. Table 17-11 presents an overview of both the normal and abnormal observations most common during functional evaluation. Occurrence of any of the abnormal responses is justification for stopping the test. The work level at which the abnormality is identified is noted to be the upper level of tolerance. Frequently, exhaustion occurs before abnormal response and functional capacity is noted at the point of exhaustion.

Reflective of ischemic conditions, the ST segment is the most closely scrutinized area of the exercise ECG. The nurse in an exercise-testing situation should be well versed in assessing this response parameter.

Currently, the most widely accepted critera for ST segment depression representative of myocardial ischemia is 1 mm. (.1mv.) or greater 80 milliseconds after the QRS-ST junction ("J" point). A four-step approach is recommended in Figure 17-5 to provide consistency in performing this ECG assessment. Figure 17-6 displays a normal exercise ST response, and Figure 17-7 shows a dramatic ST change with exercise.

Postexercise Responses

It is not uncommon for certain abnormalities to occur in the immediate poststress period even when test responses were normal. There are a significant number of patients who develop ST segment depression after exercise. The reasons are not completely understood, but are believed to be due to the sudden drop in cardiac output that may result from venous pooling in the postexercise state.[20]

Another effect of sudden venous pooling immediately upon termination of exercise is an extreme vasovagal reaction that can precipitate the heart rate from a near maximal level, such as 140 to extreme bradycardia, such as 40 in less than a minute's time.[21] This phenomenon is not considered pathologic and tends to be self-limiting as venous return stabilizes. Symptomatic support may be required in the interim.

The possibility of either of these occurrences in the postexercise state emphasizes the need for continued observation in the immediate posttest period. As soon as the test is completed, the treadmill is gradually slowed while an immediate postexercise upright ECG is recorded. The patient is then helped to sit or lie down on a nearby ECG table and subsequent postexercise responses are measured every two minutes until stable.

Table 17-10
Data Collection During Exercise Testing

Pretest	During Test		Posttest
	Each minute during test progression:	Before advancing to next stage:	Immediately and every two minutes x 3, or until stable:
Heart rate	Heart rate		Heart rate
Blood pressure		Blood pressure	Blood pressure
ECG	ECG		ECG
Signs/symptoms	Signs/symptoms		Signs/symptoms

Table 17-11
Exercise Stress Testing Response Parameters

Response	Normal	Abnormal	Abnormal Causation
Signs			
Heart rate	Increase less than ten beats per minute for each MET level of work.	A. Increase greater than ten beats per minute for each MET level of work. B. Inability of the heart rate to increase in exercise.	A. Dysfunction and/or deconditioned state. B. Chronotropic tence, drug influence (propranolol ([Inderal]).

Table 17-11
Exercise Stress Testing Response Parameters

Blood pressure	Increase of less than ten mm. systolic for each MET level of work; diastolic remains unchanged or decreases slightly.	A. Increase greater than ten mm. systolic for each MET level, or a peak B/P in excess of 250 mm. B. Failure of the systolic B/P to increase in response to exercise or decrease in systolic pressure to increasing stress.	A. Deconditioning and/or hypertensive response. B. Pump failure, iatrogenic or drug-related (proprandol [Inderal]).
ECG	Tachycardia, normal conduction; J point depression, normal ST segment.	A. ST segment depression. (1 mm or more at 80 msec. duration) B. Dysrhythmia tachycardic, bradycardic, or ectopic activity. C. Conduction defects A-V or bundle branch	A. Usually ischemic B. Frequently ischemic, although & not diagnostic unless accompanied C. By ST segment depression.
Skin signs	Pale appearance during submaximal levels due to circulatory redistribution, flushed appearance during near maximal levels due to heat buildup.	Pale or cyanotic appear-appearance late in the test.	Circulatory inadequacy
Neurological	Patient should remain alert and oriented with good psychomotor control	Loss of orientation, sudden incoordination	Decrease in cerebral flow
Symptoms			
Chest pain or discomfort	None	Any complaint of discomfort or unusual sensation in the chest, arms, neck, back, jaw, etc. should be assumed to be angina	Myocardial ischemia (pain onset may or may not correlate with ischemic ECG changes)
Dizziness, light-headedness	None	Should be assumed to be neurological symptoms	Decrease in cerebral flow
Lower extremity claudication	None	Severe muscular spasm	Frequently coexisting peripheral vascular disease
Dyspnea	Rapid breathing	Expressed difficulty breathing	Usually due to co-existing lung disease

Adapted from Ellestad, M. H., *Stress Testing, Principles and Practice*, (Philadelphia: F. A. Davis Company, 1975), p. 45; Committee on Exercise, *Exercise Testing and Training of Individuals With Heart Disease or at High Risk for Its Development: A Handbook for Physicians* (New York: American Heart Association, 1975) p. 11; and Fox, S. M., Naughton, J. P. and Haskell, W. L., "Physical Activity and Prevention of Coronary Heart Disease," *Annals of Clinical Research*, Vol. 3, 1971, pp. 404-432.

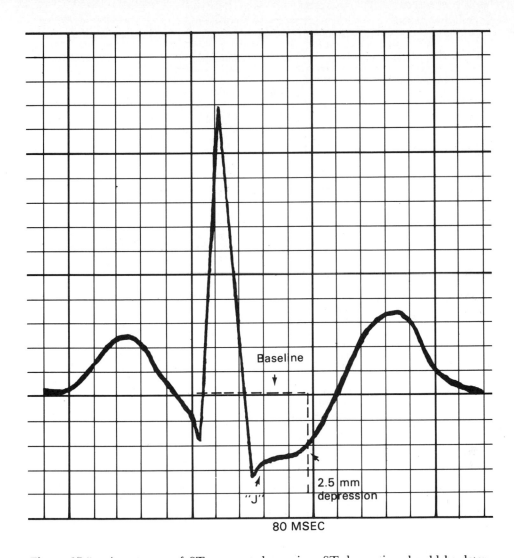

Baseline

2.5 mm depression

"J"

80 MSEC

Figure 17-5. Assessment of ST segment depression. ST depression should be deter-mined in the following manner in any lead where change is observed visually: 1. Locate a portion of the exercise ECG that is relatively free of motion artifact; establish a reference baseline, lining up the P-R intervals of three successive complexes. 2. Locate the "J" point on the middle complex; looking for the change in stylus-trace thickness from the quick, thin QRS stroke to the slower, thicker ST stroke will help pinpoint the junction. 3. Measure 80 milliseconds in a horizontal direction from the "J" point and draw a perpendicular line through the reference baseline at the measured time. 4. Measure the difference in vertical millimeters between the original baseline and the point where the ST segment intersects the time perpendicular; the number of millimeters counted is recorded as the amount of ST segment depression.

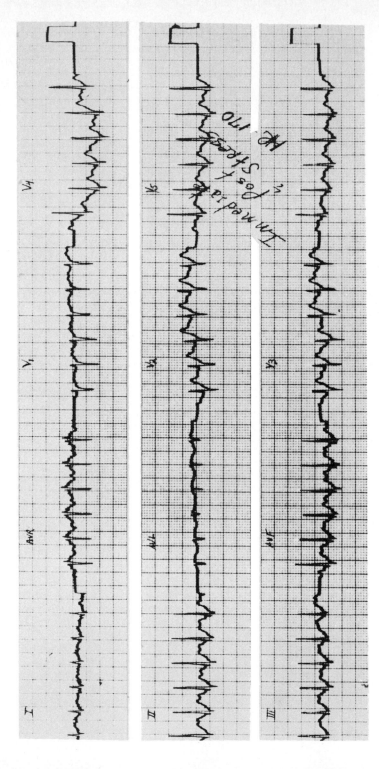

Figure 17-6. Normal ST segment response to exercise. Heart rate: 170.

Documentation

Test Results. Compilation and documentation of test data are usually the nurse's responsibility. If responses were recorded throughout the test performance (such as written on the corresponding ECG strips), it is a simple matter to transfer data onto a test report form. A report format that displays concurrent response parameters in sequential order and provides related data has proven useful. One format is shown in the sample case at the end of this chapter.

Summary and Interpretations. The physician is responsible for interpreting the test results in terms of diagnoses and/or medical therapeutics. The nurse is responsible for assessing the data and the physician's interpretation to determine problems requiring nursing intervention. Problems identified from the test should be listed under the categories of physical, psychological, and educational needs.

Physical problems emerging from an exercise stress test may include a general lack of fitness or an inability to perform safely at an energy level compatible with a previous job. Psychologically, the test may reveal that the patient has a long-held fear of exertion due to his heart condition. The problems described represent obvious health educational needs as well.

Additional needs may be determined from the physician's interpretations and/or recommendations. For example, if the patient exhibited a dysrhythmia during test performance and subsequent antidysrhythmic therapy is recommended by the physician, the patient will need to be taught the why's and how's of taking the new medication.

Direct involvement with initial exercise stress testing provides valuable assessment information for the nurse who will be working with the Phase IV cardiac rehab patient.

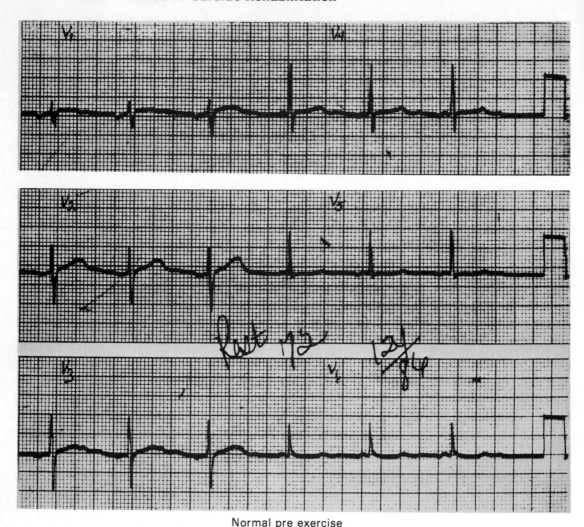

Normal pre exercise
ST segments

Figure 17-7.   Abnormal ST segment response.

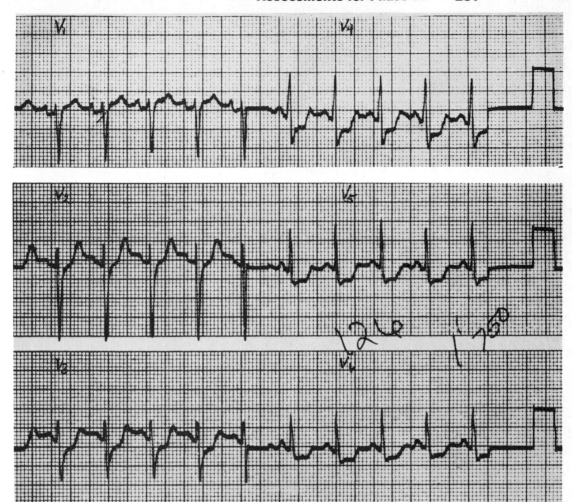

After nine minute bicycle
ergometer stress (one min.
@ 750 kpm), HR 126, 2 mm
ST segment depression in V,
"positive" test   5

(Patient ID Stamp)

C. P.	**CARDIAC REHAB PROGRESS NOTES**

Date/Time	PROGRESS NOTES
7/11/XX 10 a.m.	Phase IV admission:
	S. Patient pleased with EST performance, looking forward to doing more exercise and more farm work. "Never felt better."
	O. No abnormal pretest findings. EST responses somewhat exaggerated probably due to lack of conditioning and anxiety about test outcome. Performed 6 METS of work with no ECG abnormalities.
	A. Phase III progress reviewed. Should do well with Phase IV exercise training.
	P. Initial training session scheduled for Friday. Phase IV Rehab Plan completed.
	C. R., R.n.

(Patient ID Stamp)

C. P.

**NURSE'S
CARDIOVASCULAR
EXAMINATION**

Date   7/11/XX   **Purpose**   preceding initial EST

INSPECTION AND PALPATION:

Patient is alert, steady, has good color, and appears healthy.

Upper extremities: radial and brachial pulses regular, strong, and equal bilaterally. No edema, discoloration, or clubbing.

Chest: equal bilateral chest excursion with inspiration, normal A-P diameter. PMI at 5th ICS. No thrills.

Abdomen: flat, soft, no abnormal pulsations.

Lower extremities: popliteal and pedal pulses regular, strong, and equal bilaterally. No edema, discoloration, or varices. Neg. Homan's. Hair distribution and toenails appear normal.

AUSCULTATION:

B/P rt. arm   130/80   left arm   134/82

Heart Sounds: Apical rate at 74 and regular. No splits, gallops, murmurs, or rubs.

Lung Sounds: Respiration rate at 18. Vesicular sounds throughout lung fields. No rales, rhonchi, or rubs.

MEASUREMENT AND TESTS:

Height   5′8″   Weight   155 lbs.   Temp.   97.8 F.

Standard 12 Lead ECG:
NSR at 72, small Q's II, III, AVF-old inferior MI.

Lab Results:
CBC and electrolytes normal. Cholesterol 270 mgm% Triglycerides 146 mgm%

Chest X-ray:
Normal

C. R., R.N.

(Patient ID Stamp)

C. P.

**EXERCISE STRESS
TEST RESULTS**

Test Date ___7/11/XX___ **Time** ___8 a.m.___ **Purpose** ___initial functional evaluation___

Testing Physician ___J. D., M.D.___ **Testing Nurse** ___C. R., R.N.___

Test Device/Protocol ___Treadmill/Balke I___ **HR Guide** ___open ended, 179 PMHR___

Medications ___none___

Exercise Response Flow Chart

Work Stages	Cum. Time	Heart Rate	Blood Pressure	ST Segment	Other ECG Changes	Signs/ Symptoms
Baseline	—	74	130/80			
3 mph/0%	2	94	130/80			
3/2.5%	4	110	142/84			
3/5%	6	142	160/92			
3/7.5%	8	160	172/94	—	—	leg fatigue
Immediate		148	150/88			
2' recovery		128	144/80			
4' recovery		92	130/80			
6' recovery		84	124/74			

Reason(s) for terminating the test: ___leg fatigue___

Recorded by: ___C. R., R.N.___

(Patient ID Stamp)

C. P.

**EXERCISE STRESS TEST
PHYSICIAN'S INTERPRETATION**

7/11/XX   8:30 a.m.

TEST SUMMARY:
On this initial functional evaluation, the patient completed 8 minutes of treadmill walking before test was terminated due to leg fatigue.

Responses as follows:

HR - increase excessive per stage   }   due to lack of conditioning
B/P - also accelerated response

No ST segment depression or other ECG change.
Leg fatigue only subjective discomfort.

INTERPRETATION:
Test responses indicative of decreased fitness. Good candidate for monitored exercise training. Progressive training prescription to be written.

J. D., M.D.

References

1. BREU, C. S., "Assessment: Review of Vital Skills," *Combating Cardiovascular Diseases Skillfully* Intermed Communications Inc., Horsham, Pa., 1978, pp. 45-54.
2. ELLESTAD, M. H., *Stress Testing, Principles and Practice* (Philadelphia: F. A. Davis Company, 1975), p. 45.
3. COMMITTEE on EXERCISE, *Exercise Testing and Training of Individuals With Heart Disease or at High Risk for Its Development: A Handbook for Physicians* (New York: American Heart Association, 1975), p. 11.
4. *Ibid.*, p. 27.
5. ROCHMIS, P. and BLACKBURN, H., "Exercise Tests, A Survey of Procedures, Safety & Litigation Experience in Approximately 170,000 Tests," *JAMA*, Vol. 217, No. 8, August 1971, pp. 1061-1066.
6. TASK FORCE on CARDIOVASCULAR REHABILITATION, *Needs and Opportunities for Rehabilitating the Coronary Heart Disease Patient* (The National Heart and Lung Institute, December 1974), p. 27.
7. EXERCISE and STRESS TESTING WORKSHOP REPORT, "Exercise, Proceedings of the National Workshop on Exercise," *The Journal of the South Carolina Medical Association*, December 1969, supplement, p. 75.
8. AMERICAN COLLEGE of SPORTS MEDICINE, *Guidelines for Exercise Testing and Exercise Prescriptions* (Philadelphia: Lea & Febiger, 1975), p. 22.
9. COMMITTEE on EXERCISE, *op. cit.*, p. 18.
10. SHEFFIELD, T., et al., "Submaximal Exercise Testing," *The Journal of the South Carolina Medical Association*, December 1969, supplement, p. 21.
11. COMMITTEE on EXERCISE, *op. cit.*, p. 18.
12. ROCHMIS and BLACKBURN, *op. cit.*, pp. 1065-1066.
13. COMMITTEE on EXERCISE, *Exercise Testing and Training of Apparently Healthy Individuals: A Handbook for Physicians*, (New York: American Heart Association, 1972), p. 10.
14. HELLERSTEIN, H. K., "Exercise Tests Inadequate," *The Physician and Sports Medicine*, August 1976, p. 60.
15. ELLESTAD, *op. cit.*, p. 52.
16. *Ibid.*
17. BLACKBURN, H., et al., "Standardization of the Exercise Electrocardiogram," *Physical Activity and the Heart* (Springfield, Illinois: Charles C Thomas, 1967), pp. 101-133.
18. FROELICHER, V., et al., "A Comparison of Two Bipolar Exercise Electrocardiographic Leads to Lead V^5," *Chest*, Vol. 70, No. 5, November 1976, pp. 611-616.
19. MASON, R. E. and LIKAR, I., "A New System of Multiple Lead Exercise Electrocardiography", *American Heart Journal*, February 1966, pp. 196-205.
20. ELLESTAD, *op. cit.*, p. 115.
21. SHEFFIELD, T., "The Meaning of Exercise Test Findings," *Coronary Heart Disease: Prevention, Detection, Rehabilitation With Emphasis on Exercise Testing* (International Medical Corp., 1974).

18
planning of phase IV cardiac rehabilitation

Behavioral Objectives

After completion of this chapter, the reader should be able to:

■ identify the common nursing goals of Phase IV.

■ name the components of an exercise prescription and describe the physiological principles underlying each.

■ compare and contrast group exercise programs with exercise unit programs.

■ outline a sample sequence of events for a formal training program.

■ list at least six educational topics for which the nurse has teaching responsibility prior to a patient's home exercise program.

■ select a personal "home exercise program" to include a primary choice and at least one alternative and one adjunct of personal preference.

■ discuss the value of relaxation techniques as part of Phase IV health care.

■ discuss the value of the peer group as an educational and motivational force in a long-term program.

Introduction

In Phase IV of the cardiac rehabilitation process, as in the three preceding Phases, planning includes organizing identified needs and problems, examining available alternatives, making decisions, and identifying intentions as measurable objectives. As discussed in Chapter 16, the basic purpose of health care in Phase IV is secondary prevention. To achieve this purpose, common nursing goals based on patient similarities have been formulated (see Table 18-1).

Table 18-1
Common Nursing Goals for Phase IV Rehabilitation

Physiological

To assist the patient to attain and maintain an optimal physical state by development of training effects through a safe and effective structured exercise-training program, and maintenance of training effects through appropriate self-directed home exercise.

Psychosocial

To provide an environment which includes the professional and peer support necessary to accomplish and maintain change.
To assist the patient in developing an acceptable relaxation technique as a means of relieving normally accumulated stress.

Educational

To reinforce the awareness, skill, and affect needed for both accomplishment of Phase IV physiological/psychosocial goals and continuation of behavioral changes initiated in earlier rehab phases.

Planning lays the foundation for successful Phase IV rehabilitation. Assessment information coupled with the common nursing goals is structured into a unique rehab plan for each Phase IV patient.

Planning to Meet Physiological Goals

As a nursing goal, assisting cardiac patients to achieve their optimal level of physical function presents an original challenge with each patient. Definition of "optimal physical state" is the first planning step. In general, the optimal or best physical level for any cardiac patient is a physiological state that insofar as possible reduces future health threats from existing disease and enables the patient to conduct his daily life comfortably and realistically. Since one patient's life-style may be the direct opposite of another's, nurse and patient must work together to determine what optimal is and to construct a viable plan to achieve physiological goals.

Exercise Prescription Components

Exercise is the means by which the physiological end may be achieved. To be effective, exercise requires deliberate, knowledgeable planning. There are right ways and wrong ways for the cardiac patient to exercise. Too much exercise can be disastrous; too little may be useless.

Exercise applied to induce physiological change is a therapeutic agent and, as such, requires a physician's prescription and the informed consent of the patient. Ideally, prescription preparation and procurement of patient consent is a collaborative effort between the testing physician and the nurse specialist who will be carrying out the exercise program.

To meaningfully participate in health care decisions and to effectively plan and administer exercise therapy, the nurse must assume responsibility for knowing the principles underlying an exercise prescription, for being familiar with common prescription applications, and for knowing how program design and progression influence effectiveness.

Intensity—How Much Exercise? The right amount of exercise is the amount that sufficiently stresses the cardiovascular system to utilize adaptive mechanisms that over a period of time result in desired training effects. Research has identified a range of safe and effective cardiovascular stress between 60 to 80 percent of an individual's functional aerobic capacity as determined by exercise stress testing.[1] Therefore, exercise that produces stress levels in that range is the correct amount. Exercise performed at less than 60 percent of capacity produces little gain and, consequently, 60 percent is labeled the "training threshold." Exercise performed above 80 percent produces little added benefit and can result in unpleasant side effects or serious complications for the previously sedentary cardiac patient.[2] Obviously then, complete exercise stress test results are needed before appropriate exercise intensity can be determined.

Application. Assigning an exercise load that will produce the 60 to 80 percent aerobic response presents an application problem. Measurement of oxygen transport to determine whether or not the patient is performing in the desired range every time he exercises is both impractical and costly. Therefore, a more readily available, but equally reliable indicator of cardiovascular stress is needed to guide performance intensity. The following intensity approaches are most common:

1. The Heart Rate. The relationship between oxygen uptake and heart rate has been identified—approximately 60 to 80 percent of functional aerobic capacity is equivalent to 70 to 85 percent of maximal heart rate.[3] This equation provides a convenient method for prescribing work intensity.When one knows the maximal heart rate the individual has reached on testing, it is a simple matter to compute 70 to 85 percent of that rate. Exercise sufficient to maintain the heart rate between those limits correspondingly generates the desired aerobic performance.

   For example, a given patient is tested to maximal performance with a heart rate of 188; his effective intensity for exercise training would be a work level that produced a training heart rate (THR) between 132 (70 percent of 188) and 160 (85 percent of 188).

A formula originated by Karvonen is another popular method for determining the training rate[4]: THR = (maximum heart rate - resting heart rate) x 70% + resting rate. For example, a given patient is tested to maximal performance with a heart rate of 188; his preceding resting rate was 82: THR = (188-82) x 70% + 82 = 156.

Effective intensity for exercise training would be work that produced a training rate of 156. The advantage of this approach is that it takes into consideration the patient's resting heart rate as well as his maximal heart rate and, thus, can provide finer tuning for prescriptions.

Using the 70 to 85 percent simple computation described above, the exercise prescription may be written as an intensity *range* prescribed as: "the amount of exercise should be adjusted as necessary to keep the heart rate between 132 and 160." Or it may specify exact *targets* that progress within the limits, such as:

> week one to two exercise at a heart rate of 132 (70 percent)
> week three to four exercise at a heart rate of 141 (75 percent)
> week five to six exercise at a heart rate of 150 (80 percent)
> after six weeks, exercise at a heart rate of 160 (85 percent)

Intensity prescribed by range provides the exercise supervisor more flexibility with methods and types of exercise, while specific target prescription may provide more control.

Regardless of the method used for prescribing intensity according to heart rate, the following basic rule should always be enforced: *During exercise training, the patient's heart rate should never be allowed to exceed the maximal heart rate he demonstrated during exercise testing.* The reason, of course, is patient safety. Should the patient enter an area of untested responses, the effect cannot be anticipated.

2. The Work Level. Using available tables of standardized testing protocols equated to oxygen requirements,[5] it is a relatively easy matter to compute 60 to 80 percent of the maximal oxygen consumption from a patient's test. Converting the oxygen values to equivalent METs (3.5 ml. O_2 per minute = 1 MET) simplifies the process further. Exercise intensity can then be prescribed. For example, A given patient performs a Balke I treadmill test to a 10-MET (35 ml. oxygen per Kg. per minute) level; intensity for exercise training (60 to 80 percent aerobic capacity) would be 6 to 8 METs.

Although relatively simple to use, intensity prescribed by METs has several disadvantages: MET equivalent information is only available for a limited number of exercise-training activities; usefulness is generally restricted to standard exercise laboratory equipment. The amount of oxygen consumed (and, therefore, the number of METs used) in performing an activity is variable and can be easily altered by exercise skill, changes in psychological state, and environment; the prescription, therefore, may not be consistently reproducible.

3. Subjective Intensity. The methods described above provide objective means of controlling exercise training so that it is both effective and

safe. Although many patients do come to "feel" when the amount of exercise is appropriate, subjective sensations should not be solely relied on to guide intensity of performance with cardiac patients. Instructions like "exercise until you perspire . . . until you feel tired . . ." may be useful as warning signs in some cases, but should always be supplemented by heart rate determination.

Duration—How Long? In order to achieve the desired training effects, an exerciser must not only reach his prescribed training intensity (heart rate), but must continue the work to sustain the training level for a period of time. Thirty-minute exercise sessions are suggested for optimal effectiveness.[6] Most programs use a duration range of 20 to 40 minutes performance at prescribed intensity.

Application. The complete exercise-training session is composed of three separately timed parts, each having a distinct purpose:

1. The Warm-up Segment. Usually five to ten minutes long, the warm-up consists of low-level activity performed to stimulate circulatory and respiratory adjustments, to loosen joints and muscles and to reduce strain, to increase body and muscle temperature ("warm-up") and, thus, to enhance metabolic reactions associated with higher-level exercise.[7] Warm-up can be accomplished through use of flexibility exercises and cardiac calisthenics as performed in Phase III.

   These calisthenics should be performed energetically enough to accomplish the purposes of warm-up, but not too vigorously to overaccelerate the heart rate. Generally, the heart rate generated by warm-up should be about halfway between resting and prescribed exercise target.

   As part of the cardiac rehab team, a physical therapist or physical educator can be helpful in recommending any number of flexibility exercises or variations of those most common. As patients progress in exercise training, the addition of light resistance, such as hand dumbbells, might be considered with the warm-up exercises.

2. The Training Segment. Length of the training segment corresponds to the prescribed exercise duration. In other words, it is the duration of the training segment that is prescribed, while other parts of the session require "extra" time.

   The training segment may be conducted in either of two ways:

   Interval training is a series of repeated bouts of exercise alternated with periods of relief.[8] As usually applied to exercise training in cardiac rehabilitation, interval training employs work intervals of three to five minutes duration, followed by a relief period. The intervals are repeated as many times as necessary to complete the prescribed duration, accumulating only work interval time in the performance total. Time between work intervals is labeled the relief interval and is generally as long as the work segment (three to five minutes). It would not be appropriate to label this component as a rest interval, since during this time low-level activity, such as walking or flexibility exercises, is recommended.

Since most cardiac patients beginning exercise training were previously sedentary and perhaps recently on enforced bed rest, muscular fatigue is common. Interval training offers the advantage of enabling the patient to achieve higher levels of work briefly without undue muscle strain. Providing the exerciser with this ability can be a psychological as well as a physical boost. In addition, interval training correlates well with work tasks and daily activities that occasionally require higher levels of physical performance for short periods.

As the name implies, *continuous training* is exercise that is performed without interruption. It is commonly called endurance training. The intent of endurance training is to stimulate the oxygen transport system until a "steady state" is reached.[9] The steady state is the point at which a physiological balance between the oxygen demand of exercise and the oxygen supplied via adaptive mechanisms is demonstrated by stabilization of increased responses, including heart rate, blood pressure, and respiration.

When performing a given work level, it takes most exercisers two to three minutes until the oxygen demand and supply reach a steady state.[10] If muscular strength is adequate and if all other conditions remain constant, the steady state can be continued uninterrupted for the total training duration. Continuous training provides the advantage of being adaptable to many sport and recreational activities.

As previously described, the exercise intensity is a work level that produces a heart rate response between 70 to 85 percent of the maximal rate demonstrated on exercise testing. In carrying out the training segment, it is important to realize that there is an inverse relationship between the exercise intensity and the exercise duration.[11]

For example, if exercise intensity was prescribed as 85 percent accumulating 20 minutes of interval exercise performance would be appropriate. The patient would most likely be able to perform the high corresponding work level for three- to five-minute periods if interspersed with relief. Conversely, if prolonged exercise such as 30 to 40 minutes performance was desirable, intensity would need to be prescribed at the low end of the range (70 percent).

In practice, the two approaches (interval and continuous) frequently melt together as training progresses. Due to lack of muscular strength early in a training program, many patients are started exercising using the interval approach with a 1:1 work-relief ratio. As strength develops, the work interval time may be lengthened and the relief interval time may be shortened. A six-minute work interval with a three-minute relief interval is not uncommon. See Figure 18-1 for a graphic display of interval and continuous applications.

3. The Cool-down Segment. Following performance of the prescribed exercise intensity for the prescribed exercise duration, a period of physiological readjustment to a nonexercise state is necessary. The purpose of this immediate postexercise cool-down is to avoid venous

pooling and its accompanying side effects.

The cool-down usually consists of light activity, such as walking and deep breathing performed for five to ten minutes.

Frequency—How Often? In order for training effects to develop, the appropriate exercise intensity must be performed for the appropriate duration three to four times per week.[12]

Application. Once the frequency of training is prescribed, scheduling of the exercise sessions should be arranged. Nonconsecutive days are recommended. At the convenience of the patient, using the minimum frequency of three times per week, exercise may be scheduled for Monday, Wednesday, and Friday, or Tuesday, Thursday, and Saturday sessions. Establishing specific "exercise days" helps develop the habit of exercise.

An additional frequency consideration is that of training "maintenance." That is, once training effects have been achieved, how often must exercise be repeated in order to maintain the training level? The relationship between frequency and duration greatly influences training maintenance. Assuming that intensity is appropriate, either three twenty-minute exercise sessions, or two thirty-minute sessions would maintain the achieved fitness level.[13]

If training is discontinued, the benefits gained decline rapidly. As much as half of the training effects are lost in five weeks if training does not resume.[14]

Type—What Kind? For safe and effective cardiovascular conditioning, exercise must be aerobic, isotonic, and submaximal. As discussed in Chapter 16, aerobic indicates that sufficient oxygen is being taken in, transported, and used for the exercise performance. Isotonic exercise involves rhythmic activity of major muscle groups. Submaximal exercise is defined by the intensity prescribed between 70 to 85 percent of the maximal work achievement on exercise testing.

When the exercise prescription fulfills the criteria for intensity, duration, frequency, and general type of exercise, any specific exercise may be recommended.[15] Walking, jogging, running, cycling, rowing, swimming, jumping rope, dancing, or calisthenics used independently or in combinations are all effective training modes. These activities are commonly recommended since they do not require a high degree of psychomotor skill, such as may be required for the use of sport-related training activities (for example, basketball).

Since optimal training effects are the goal, the exercises planned should provide for meaningful muscular conditioning as well as cardiovascular training. Alternate use of leg muscles and arm muscles for training provides cardiovascular conditioning as well as skeletal muscle strengthening useful in a variety of daily activities. In other words, the primary cardiovascular effect can be gained through either leg or arm work. Muscle strengthening is a secondary gain. Leg muscle training may be useful to the patient for activities that involve walking or running actions. Arm muscle training may be specifically useful for activities such as lifting, pulling, reaching, and the like, many of which may be job-related. Offering both leg and arm work provides a well-rounded program.

Summary. With this background information in mind and with the patient's exercise test results in hand, physician and nurse can complete the exercise prescription. Review of other assessment data is essential at this point to double

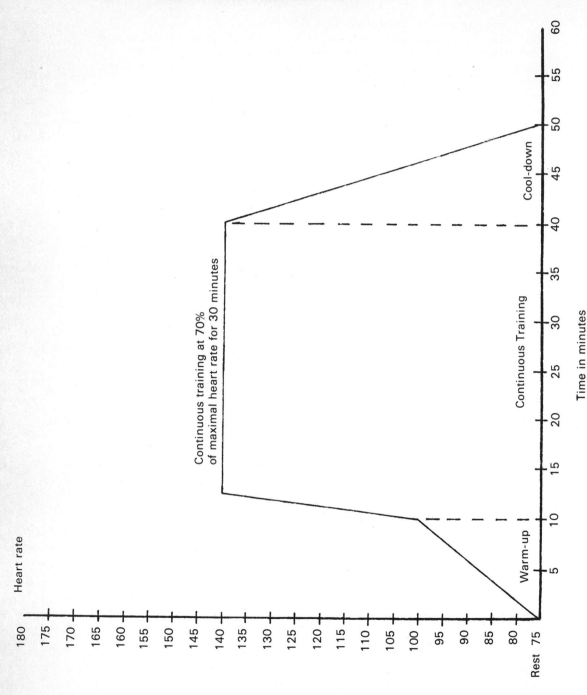

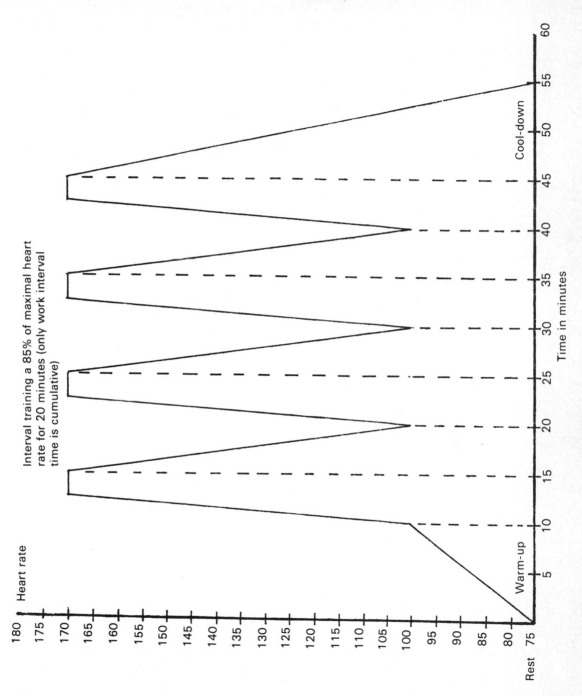

Interval training a 85% of maximal heart rate for 20 minutes (only work interval time is cumulative)

Heart rate

Time in minutes

check that there is no evidence of existing contraindications to exercise (see Chapter 16) and that other physical limitations have been considered and the prescription modified accordingly. A sample exercise prescription is included in the chapter summary.

Planning includes anticipating future needs as well as solving present problems. No therapy is effective indefinitely, including the best-planned exercise. Prescriptions must be reviewed periodically and revised as necessary to assure continued effectiveness. The most precise way to determine continuing relevance of a prescription and to home in on changes that may be necessary is to retest the patient. Planning ahead to retest the patient approximately every six weeks as recommended by the American Heart Association in the early months of a training program[16] will provide standard prescription checkpoints.

Exercise Program Design

Planning to administer an exercise prescription is obviously influenced by the design of the exercise program at hand. Internal program design is influenced by many factors, including sponsor philosophy, space availability, financial resources, and personnel training. The following are major design alternatives with which the rehab nurse should be familiar:

Unsupervised vs. Supervised Programs. As the term implies, an *unsupervised program* is one in which the patient performs exercise without direct professional assistance. Such a program may be self-initiated without definitive guidelines or may be the self-directed implementation of an exercise prescription. Unsupervised programs are discouraged for anyone beginning an exercise program except the young known healthy individual, and even then these programs should not be undertaken without official exercise testing and prescription.

In contrast, *supervised programs* provide experienced professionals to observe, advise, and assess exercise performance as defined by physician prescription. All cardiac patients should begin exercise training in a supervised setting.

Supervised programs can be further defined as being monitored or unmonitored.

1. Monitored exercise. Technology has provided exercise supervisors with the means of precise, instant performance evaluation.

   Exercise performance using telemetry ECG monitoring provides both valuable heart rate data and constant ECG evaluation (see Chapter 14 for an illustration of telemetry use).

   A variety of devices that measure, display, and/or sound the pulse rate are available. In the absence of telemetry, these may be advantageous during early weeks of training when patients are not yet proficient in pulse taking or during complicated exercises when manual pulse taking is not feasible.

   Cost, space confinement, and potential device dependency are negative aspects that must be dealt with when considering program monitoring.

2. Unmonitored Exercise. Exercise without electronic aids relies heavily on manual measurement of the exercise pulse to guide performance. Therefore, greater margin of error is possible. Self-reliance and unlimited application of manual heart rate assessment are assets.
3. In-between Approaches. Intermittent monitoring is an adaptation of ECG monitoring that has been useful in some programs. Each exercising patient has his ECG "checked" from time to time during the session, usually through the use of the monitoring paddles of a defibrillator. One disadvantage of this approach is that it does not capture the ECG at the peak of exercise performance.

Some programs decide which patients need to be monitored and which do not on an individualized basis. If this approach is utilized, well-defined medical criteria are required to assure that appropriate patients are monitored. For example, the "to be monitored" group might include any patient who exhibited dysrhythmia on exercise testing, any patient who experienced chest pain during testing, any patient who has a family history of sudden cardiac death, and so on.

Group Sport Programs vs. Exercise Unit Programs. Carried out in a gym setting, the *group sport* approach readily accommodates a large group of exercisers. In its simplest form, it may include a combination of group calisthenics, walking, and jogging performance. Greater diversity may be added by including sports such as volleyball or basketball, and where available, swimming. Depending on location and weather conditions, the "gym class" may be held outdoors and may include use of a track for jogging.

With *the exercise unit* approach, training sessions are conducted in structured exercise units, usually consisting of several adjustable, preferably calibrated, exercise appliances. Sophisticated units may have as many as six to eight "exercise stations" such as bicycle ergometers, treadmills, stepping benches, and jump ropes for leg work; wall pulleys, arm ergometers, rowing machines, and punching bags for arm work. The exerciser would rotate work performance among the appliances. Figure 18-2 illustrates simple and sophisticated exercise unit possibilities.

A summary of advantages and disadvantages of each approach is presented in Table 18-2.

A community in which both programs are available and work in cooperation is probably the ideal. Patients could then be referred to the program that is most appropriate for their condition and preference. Introduction of an "exercise shuttle"—alternating group and unit programs—might provide cumulative advantage to selected patients.

Exercise-Training Progression

Given an exercise prescription that fulfills the principles previously described and given a functional program design, planning must next consider what sequence of events is appropriate for an exercise-training program. Initially, the patient will require direction—what to do and how to do it—labeled the dependent segment. With good teaching and some experience, the patient will

Table 18-2
Exercise Program Design Advantages/Disadvantages

	Advantages	Disadvantages
Group Sport Programs	Provide more variety and may enhance motivation Easily result in group identification and mutual support benefits Activities are directly applicable to many familiar activities and, thus, may result in a smoother transition to home exercise Less cost to patient	Large groups can dilute individual supervision. Group programs tend to be unmonitored (cost of monitoring the total group would be prohibitive, selective or intermittent monitoring may be useful). Games may require some degree of psychomotor skill not necessarily possessed by a previously sedentary individual; discouragement may result. Times when the gym may be used for cardiac exercise class may be restricted and inconvenient for many. Games may stimulate competitive drives in spite of efforts to reduce this added psychological stress.
Exercise Unit Programs	Provide individualized supervision Offer convenience and flexibility of individual exercise appointments Monitoring devices can be effectively utilized Responses can be more closely controlled and reproduced due to equipment settings Equipment use does not require any special skill; with simple instruction and demonstration, it can be used effectively Structured approach and individualized attention may enhance motivation	Exercise appliances may not be easily available (or affordable) for home use. Boredom due to confinement is a possibility. Greater cost to patient

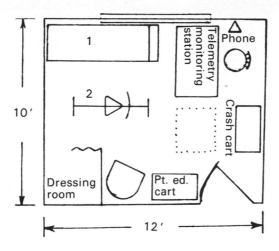

Simple exercise unit

Total space 120 sq. ft.

Exercise stations

1. Treadmill

2. Bicycle ergometer

Dotted area shows space available
for warm-up and cool-down exercises

Figure 18-2. A sophisticated exercise unit.

progress to the point where he needs coaching—helpful reminders and correction of mistakes—labeled the transition segment. Before long, the patient will need only occasional advice—assistance when new or unusual circumstances arise—labeled the independent segment. Anticipating and preparing for this progression is a major planning responsibility.

The Dependent Segment. As mentioned previously, exercise for every cardiac patient should be supervised. The guidance of a knowledgeable exercise supervisor in the initial weeks of a training program is essential to safety and effectiveness.

The question of how long direct supervision should continue does not have an absolute answer. The end of the dependent segment of an exercise program is a function of physiology rather than chronology. That is, progression into the next segment results from evidence of improvement and capability to continue under self-direction, not just from the passage of time.

The extent to which individuals develop physiological improvements as a result of exercise training varies from person to person. In like manner, the rate at which the training effects develop varies. Most faithful exercise participants begin to exhibit improved function after six to ten weeks of training.[17] Twenty to thirty weeks may be needed to achieve optimal training in some individuals.[18]

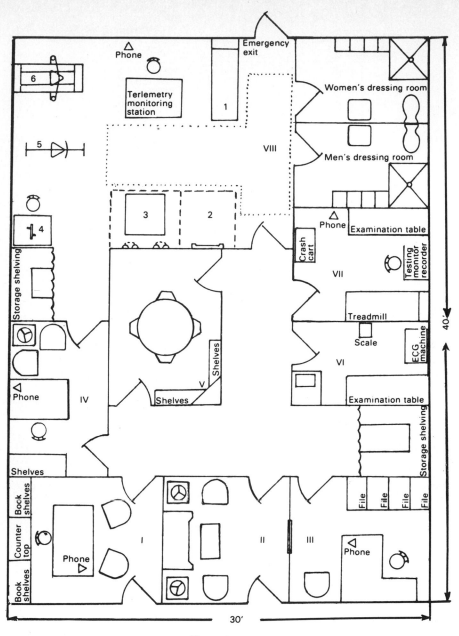

Phone

Terlemetry monitoring station

6

5

4

Storage shelving

Phone

IV

Shelves

Shelves

Book shelves

Counter top

Book shelves

Phone

I

3

2

V

Shelves

II

III

Phone

Emergency exit

1

VIII

Women's dressing room

Men's dressing room

Phone   Examination table

Crash cart

VII

Testing monitor recorder

Treadmill

Scale

ECG machine

VI

Examination table

Storage shelving

File File File File

40'

30'

Main entrance

Sophisticated exercise unit
Total space 1200 sq. ft.
I. Medical director's office
II. Reception/waiting
III. Clerical office
IV. Nurse coordinator's office

V. Educational/counseling room
VI. Examination room
VII. Exercise testing room
VIII. Exercise training room
Exercise stations
1. Treadmill

2. Wall pulleys
3. Jumping ropes
4. Arm ergometer
5. Bicycle ergometer
6. Rowing machine
Dotted area shows space available
for warm-up and cool-down exercises

270

	M T W Th F S	M T W Th F S	M T W Th F S	M T W Th F S	M T W Th F S	M T W Th F S	M T W Th F S	M T W Th F S
EST #1	X X	X X X X	X X X X X X	X X X X X X	X X X X X X	X X X X X X	X X X X X X	X X X X X X
EST #2	X X	X X X X	X X X X X X	X X X X X X	X X X X X X	X X X X X X	X X X X X X	X X X X X X
EST #3	X X	X X X H	X X X X X H	X X X X X H	X X X X X H	X X X X X H	X X X X X H	H X H X X H
EST #4	H X	H X H X H H	H H H H H H	H H H H H H	H H H H H H	H H H H H H	H H H H H H	H X H X X H
EST #5	Continue home exercise 3X wk. Schedule periodic "check-up" visits
EST #6	6 months after #5. Repeat testing annually thereafter

Dependent segment

Transition segment

Independent segment

X - Supervised exercise visits

H - Home exericse performance

EST - Exercise stress test

Figure 18-3. Basic training plan.

Because of such response variability, ideal length for a supervised program is difficult to establish. But, as in any long-term health program, some format is needed to guide progression. One approach that provides a general working structure while still leaving room for individual flexibility is the use of a "basic training program."

As illustrated in Figure 18-3, this mapped-out progression provides a twelve-week supervised exercise program, building in the prescribed training frequency of three times per week and the recommended serial-testing frequency of every six weeks. The twelve-week supervised structure works well with most patients, but there are exceptions. Some patients may progress rapidly and not require supervision that often for that long, while others may have limitations that hinder achievement within that time frame. The basic training plan is simply a reference guide, not a treatment rule, and the supervised segment should be shortened or lengthened according to each patient's progress.

Once the length of the dependent (supervised) program is selected, preparation for the next segment of exercise progression gets into full swing. In fact, home exercise program preparation actually begins with the first meeting between nurse and patient—the admission interview. The patient should know at the outset that responsibility for his exercise program will gradually be transferred to him. As training progresses through the dependent segment, patient and nurse discuss home exercise arrangements and plan ahead.

The science of planning home exercise is relatively simple—the same principles must be followed at home as were strictly enforced in the structured setting. The art of home exercise planning presents a vast challenge. The number of home exercise requests is only limited by the number of patients participating in the exercise program.

The task of planning home exercise can be eased and organized for both nurse and patient if it is appproached in three parts: primary program, alternatives, and adjuncts.

The Primary Home Exercise Program. A list of exercise choices that could fulfill all the principles of exercise prescription if properly carried out at home should be prepared by the nurse. For example, home exercise choices may include stationary bicycle, swimming, jogging, cycling, jumping rope, or group activities at the community center. The list should reflect the more common choices that have proven successful, but should not exclude other possibilities in special cases (see Table 18-3).

The choices should be reviewed with the patient and his other preferences added and discussed in like manner. Selection of a primary program is the patient's decision. The nurse functions as an advisor and educator, teaching proper performance of the activities and discussing the advantages and disadvantages to be considered.

Home Exercise Alternatives. Home exercise planning should include identification and discussion of recreational and sport activities that can be substituted for the primary program. Doubles tennis and basketball are examples of substitute activities that many patients enjoy, but simply wouldn't be able to do often enough to fulfill the prescription frequency. Encouraging use of such activities as available will provide variety and enhance exercise motivation.

Table 18-3
Primary Home Exercise Program Suggestions

Activity	Pros to Ponder	Cons to Consider
Calibrated bicycle ergometer	Already familiar to patients trained in exercise units; intensity easy to apply and reproduce; an appliance at home will be a tangible reminder of the importance of exercise.	Can the patient afford it? Does he have space at home? Will he persist in using it indefinitely or will early boredom occur if another alternative is not provided?
Cycling	Outdoor bicycle riding can provide scenic variety and aesthetic as well as physical stimulation; can be a family event.	Where does the patient live? What is the terrain? How often will weather interfere?
Jogging	Readily available to most patients at little cost (proper shoes are a necessity); can be a family or group event.	Investigate the same questions as with cycling, plus: how self-motivated is the patient? How many excuses will the patient find for not jogging as scheduled?
Jumping rope	Can be made available at little cost; can be done without leaving home.	What alternatives can be arranged to prevent boredom? Is there adequate jumping space in the patient's house or yard?
Stationary bicycle	Less costly than an ergometer, but no measurable intensity; still provides an appliance reminder; excellent bad weather alternative for primary outdoor program.	Will the patient persist if used as primary program?
Swimming	Excellent exercise that can be family fun; training use dependent upon method of swimming.	How available is the pool? If outdoor, will the patient go there often enough?

Adjuncts to Home Exercise. Discussion of activities that are *not* substitutes for home exercise is equally important. Activities like bowling or golf, although preferred by many patients, are not vigorous enough to generate training heart rates for an appropriate period of time. As long as there are no other limiting factors, such as heat and humidity, these activities are usually allowed at this rehab stage but are considered additions to, rather than part of, the home exercise program. The physical educator or exercise physiologist is a valuable resource to be consulted when questions arise or when unusual requests are encountered in planning home programs.

The Transition Segment. As previously described, the dependent program segment does not just come to a dead end. Instead, the patient is gradually weaned from professional control and supervision to independent management. Two factors contribute to the decision to begin weaning: physiological improvement as demonstrated on repeat exercise stress test (see Chapter 20 for discussion of evaluation parameters) and psychological readiness to accept the responsibility for health maintenance.

The first factor is an objective measurement and, therefore, can be well defined. If the patient shows evidence of improvement and has had no adverse effects to the supervised exercise therapy, he is likely to proceed through transition. The second factor is the combined subjective opinion of the nurse and patient, obviously less definitive. Experience is the best aid to judging readiness.

"Weaning" must be planned in advance and involves gradually transferring one visit per week from the controlled environment to home. The patient should select which of the three exercise days he would like to perform at home instead of at the exercise facility. The other two days he will continue to come to the supervised sessions. These sessions will be used to discuss his home exercise and offer guidance as needed. This two-day-in/one-day-out step should last three to four weeks. The next weaning step is the reverse. One day in/two days out. Again, three to four weeks is suggested.

The Independent Segment—Lifelong Maintenance. And now—graduation. All planning to meet physiological goals is ultimately directed toward this end—maintenance of optimal physical health, self-directed by the patient. Independence does not mean total discontinuation of professional assistance. Before entering this segment, a follow-up system is arranged—check-up visits, phone calls, and so on. The patient should be assured that he has an ongoing professional contact (see Chapter 20 for discharge discussion). Figure 18-3 delineates the three successive segments of a basic training program.

Planning to Meet Psychosocial Goals

Comprehensive cardiac rehabilitation involves assisting the patient to achieve an optimal level of well-being psychosocially as well as physically. As defined and detailed in previous phases, psychosocial considerations deal with the patient and his usual environment and relationships. Social, vocational, and psychological concerns may all be placed in this category.

The groundwork for optimizing psychosocial status was laid early in the rehab process and was progressively built upon during the three preceding rehab phases. It remains for the nurse in Phase IV to assure that the patient is in a life position that is meaningful to him.

Interpersonal Relations

Work life, home life, and sex life should be approaching a level that is functional and acceptable to the patient as he enters Phase IV. Concentrated efforts were made in Phase III to prevent relationship problems that commonly occur with postacute cardiac patients, but there is no guarantee that such nursing prophylaxis will be effective in all cases. Thus, the necessity for planning to assist the patient to achieve satisfactory relationships in Phase IV.

Two assumptions are made in this part of the planning process: first, that the majority of patients will be well on their way to re-establishing old or building new relationships, but that progress may be enhanced and the number of backslidings reduced if professional and peer support is readily available.

Second, that an occasional patient will have a serious psychological problem that hinders relationship development in spite of earlier rehab efforts. With these two possibilities in mind, the Phase IV nurse must be prepared to act as group coordinator and/or professional liaison.

Coordinator. One of the biggest advantages of a formal outpatient cardiac rehab program is that it provides two effective support mechanisms for the patient evolving through the postcardiac period:

1. Frequent, consistent professional contact—the patient can share information, ask questions, and discuss problems with a nurse he has learned is knowledgeable and caring.

2. Group process can be employed by the skillful nurse to give peer support to a concerned patient and peer approval to patients who have achieved desirable outcomes. The "peers," of course, are other cardiac patients. The supportive role of the group can be subtly elicited in conjunction with a group function organized for another purpose, such as an educational program, or the group may be held specifically to provide a forum for problem discussion. In the latter case, the nurse should maintain the group on an expressive, problem-solving level. Analytical levels, more typical of psychotherapy groups, should not be attempted without the presence of a qualified psychologist.

Liaison. If an apparent psychological problem or relationship crisis has been identified either through history update, spontaneous information from the patient, or investigation of behavioral change, immediate planning should involve contacting the appropriate professional specialst. Specialists frequently consulted during Phase IV rehab include the psychologist or psychological social worker, the family therapist, the sex therapist, the vocational rehab counselor, and the occupational therapist.

Simple discussion of the problem may provide the rehab nurse with an insight or suggestion she needs to further plan how to assist the patient. The other possibility is that the nurse will discover that the problem could be more serious than superficially indicated and that referral should be made for formal counseling. Depending upon the nature of the problem and the policies of the institutions involved, referral may require a physician's order.

Personal Relaxation

According to Hans Selye, "In its medical sense, stress is essentially the rate of wear and tear in the body. For scientific purposes, stress is defined as the state which manifests itself by the General Adaptation Syndrome . . . adrenal stimulation, shrinkage of lymphatic organs, gastrointestinal ulcers, loss of body weight, alterations in the chemical composition of the body, and so forth."[19] Teaching cardiac patients about stress is a routine part of the inpatient educational program. Advising patients to review their life priorities is a standard part of postdischarge counseling. But frequently, it is not until the patient has resumed his normal daily activities that he is aware of what all the warnings meant. Once again, daily stress and strain are upon him. This stress realization generally coincides with Phase IV rehab. Anticipating the need for stress-reduction assistance, planning should consider what alternatives the Phase IV nurse can suggest.

Table 18-4
Stress Reduction Techniques

Type	Description	Performance	Advantages
Autogenic training	Self-generated and self-controlled relaxation; initial professional instruction may be needed to acquaint an individual or group with the method.	Autosuggestion is used to achieve the relaxed state. The person selects his preferred point of concentration. The following approaches have been used successfully: Rhythm concentration 1. Breathing provides a readily available rhythm......in.......out...... 2. Counting Forward or backward at a soothing cadence or in time with breathing. 3. A soothing word or phrase ......one....one....one.... ......love...love...love.... ......I am..I am...I am.... NOTE: Words are not spoken out loud but occur in the mind. Sensation concentration A change of sensation is accomplished by concentrating on successive muscle groups or parts of the body, beginning at either the head or the feet. 1. Muscle relaxation All voluntary effort is concentrated on relaxing the part. 2. Warmth and heaviness All thoughts are focused on achieving a warm, heavy feeling in the respective part. Imagery concentration 1. Imagining a favorite tranquil scene and concentrating on being there: the beach at sunset, a mountain lake. 2. Imagining a peaceful descent from a place of high activity to one of quiet and rest: as on a long, slow escalator or a cable car.	Once learned and practiced, the technique can be applied as needed in a variety of daily situations.

Biofeedback	The use of physiological measurements to train voluntary control of autonomic responses such as heart rate, blood pressure, and muscle tension	The individual is connected to an appropriate monitoring instrument (ECG, EMG, etc.) and told to concentrate on the specific response being trained. Measurements made by the machine encourage the individual to intensify his efforts until the desired response ia achieved. Achievement feedback is frequently given by visual or auditory signal.	Provides an objective measurement of success
Transcendental meditation	Advanced levels of autogenic relaxation practiced to achieve the higher goal of mind expansion, usually in conjunction with a philosophical or religious belief	A word or phrase called a 'mantra' is silently repeated to quiet the body and still the mind.	The possibility of a "mystical" experience is attractive and can be an effective motivator for participation.
Yoga		Concentration on a physical or mental object is used to attain a deep meditative state. A specific posture is used to control the body.	

Adapted from Brown, B., *Stress & the Art of Biofeedback* (New York: Harper & Row, Publishers, Inc., 1977); Benson H., *The Relaxation Response* (New York: Avon Publishers, Inc., 1975); and Pelletier, K., *Mind as Healer, Mind as Slayer* (New York: Dell Publishing Co., 1977).

Many stress reduction techniques are currently in vogue although the benefits of planned relaxation have yet to be documented in scientific detail. Which method is used with a given patient is generally a matter of availability and personal preference. No one is necessarily more effective than another, although a patient may need to try several before finding one that works for him and with which he is comfortable. A descriptive outline of various techniques is presented in Table 18-4.

Regardless of the technique that is chosen, the following principles are generally employed:

- Find a quiet place in which to relax where disturbances are unlikely to occur.
- Adopt a passive attitude—trying too hard to make relaxation work will be a source of stress in itself; try to "not care" if it works or not, just relax and feel good about having had the time of no activity.
- Assume a comfortable position, but not one likely to promote sleep. Sitting, hands resting in the lap and feet placed comfortably on the floor may work for most patients.

The goal of relaxation techniques is to give body systems a rest period from accelerated responses and, eventually, to train the body to recognize stress symptoms and voluntarily counteract them. Just as the effects of the "flight or fight" reaction continue for a period of time after crisis has passed, so too the responses of relaxation carry into the active period that follows. Benson describes results of blood pressure decreases which persist from day to day as patients participate in relaxation techniques on a regular basis.[20]

CAUTION relaxation techniques are not a substitute for professional counseling and should not be suggested for patients in whom a psychological or psychiatric disturbance is suspected.

Planning to Meet Educational Goals

Education has been an essential part of the rehab process since the patient was admitted as an acute cardiac. Beginning with bedside exchanges among nurse, patient, and significant others, the teaching/learning process advanced through lessons constructed to meet patient and family learning needs in preparation for discharge. In Phase III, educational efforts continued with emphasis on teaching the patient how to specifically use his newly acquired health information in his daily life.

Applying Specific Knowledge

Much of the patient's previously learned health knowledge converges in Phase IV to be applied to the transfer of exercise responsibility from supervised setting to home. The nurse assesses each patient's educational readiness prior to home exercise approval. An assessment tool (see Table 18-5) can be helpful in determining the patient's knowledge level.

Table 18-5
Educational Assessment in Preparation for Home Exercise Initiation

---

To safely and effectively conduct an independent exercise program, the patient must be able to:

State his prescribed training heart rate (THR).

Correctly demonstrate how to take his exercise pulse.

Outline his home exercise schedule, including correct frequency and duration.

Name his choice of primary home programs.

Correctly demonstrate (if physically possible in supervised setting, otherwise describe) performance of the primary program.

Describe corrective actions to be taken if exercise pulse is above or below THR.

Discuss precautions to be taken with exercise training, including environment, clothing, and food.

Name at least one alternative method of exercise that may be substituted for the primary program.

Describe a plan of action in the event of unusual exercise effects.

Display some method of recording home exercise responses and progress.

Planning for Phase IV education, therefore, emphasizes evaluation of earlier learning so that misconceptions can be clarified and knowledge pertinent to physiological goals can be reinforced. Occasionally, a patient will enter Phase IV without benefit of previous health teaching and, in that case, a total cardiac education program will need to be planned.

Enhancing General Awareness

As discussed in earlier phases, groups can provide an effective means of reinforcing cognitive information as well as maintaining the affect essential to behavioral change and therapeutic compliance.

The Informal Group. One of the best educational tools available to the Phase IV nurse is the informal patient group. Patients who are exercising in a group will frequently be heard "educating each other." Alert nurses can capitalize on this spontaneity. A patient may benefit more from hearing a fellow patient describe how he handled a crisis or was able to achieve desirable behavior than from repeated admonitons from the nurse. For example, the nurse may ask an experienced patient to describe the use of a mutually prescribed medication to a new patient. This technique has an advantage for each patient: a "voice of experience" from a respected peer for the patient-learner, an opportunity for the nurse to evaluate the knowledge level of the patient-teacher.

The Planned Group. In planning group educational events, the nurse should review the value of each of the following group options:

1. A general group program with an open invitation to all outpatients, their familites, and friends. For example, a program on "Nutrition and Cardiac Health."

2. A subgroup program, such as, only for patients. Patients are frequently more opem in discussing their sexual concerns among their peers than in a group including spouses.

Only for spouses. Husbands or wives are more likely to discuss their fears of a spouse's sudden death without the spouse present.

Only for patients with a particular problem. The smoking and overweight groups are examples.

The Community Group A number of groups have developed around the needs of postacute cardiac patients for mutual involvement, support, and continuing education. In planning for the time when the patient will complete his structured program, the Phase IV nurse should know which cardiac-related groups are available in the community and what their respective purposes are. Appropriate patients can then be referred to the group for additional educational reinforcement and group support of their health efforts.

If a patient group is not already available, the nurse may take up the challenge of organizing a "Graduate Cardiac Club" (see Table 18-6). The self-propagation of such a graduate group is in itself a testimony of successful rehabilitation.

Table 18-6
Helpful Hints for Organizing a Graduate Cardiac Club

1. Organize a small planning committee to include an equal number of health professionals and cardiac patients.
2. Seek sponsorship: a local health agency, a hospital, or a civic group, (mainly to provide clerical assistance).
3. Find a location (free of charge) to accommodate meetings.
4. Conduct a preliminary survey of patients to determine desired frequency of meetings and topics of interest. Select educational topics and possible speakers (free of charge).
5. Draft a meeting schedule — dates and times. Allow time for an educational program and socializing at each meeting.
6. Advertise (as free) and promote first program to recruit members. Membership is voluntary and free.
7. Plan election of "officers" after several meetings and designate responsibilities, such as: 1st Officer—conduct meetings; contact rehab "graduates" or other cardiac patients to extend membership invitation; 2nd Officer—organize programs and handle meeting arrangements; 3rd Officer—keep list of members and record of programs and work with sponsor in distributing notices. A professional advisor should also be elected or appointed.

Finalizing the Plan

So far, planning has been a mental endeavor—the nurse synthesizing the principles to be followed and the means available to pursue Phase IV goals into viable alternatives. Planning now becomes synonymous with communication. A planning conference is scheduled to include the nurse, the patient, and significant others for the purpose of reviewing the needs and problems identified and offering the alternatives for corrective-preventive action.

Recalling the definition of cardiac rehabilitation, ". . . the active process of assisting the patient . . . ," the nurse should remind herself that rehab decisions belong to the patient. The patient has the right to accept or reject alternatives and to define the exact terms of the plan. The nurse is simply an advisory agent providing explanation and clarification so that the patient can make informed decisions.

Giving the patient responsibility for health care, such as long-term cardiac rehabilitation, has risks. What the patient chooses to do may not coincide with what the nurse would like to do for him. Accepting the patient's decisions under such circumstances can be the most difficult of professional tasks.

Once the patient has expressed his intentions, it remains for the nurse to transcribe his decisions into the form of behavioral objectives (see Chapter 8). Documentation of the objectives on the care plan implies that a commitment has been made between nurse and patient on behalf of the patient's present and future health and that mutual efforts to achieve the stated aims are underway.

(Patient ID Stamp)

C. P.

**CARDIAC REHAB
CARE PLAN**

Date Identified	Need/Problem	Approach	Behavioral Objectives	Date Achieved Changed
7/11/XX	**Physiological**		The patient will be able to	
	1. low fitness level	1. a) implement Phase IV exercise train-	1. show evidence of improving fitness through lower heart rate and	
		ing program per prescription	B/P responses to submax. work levels on 2nd and 3rd EST	
		b) explain the possible benefits of		
		consistent exercise		
	Psychosocial			
	2. tends to overdo has difficulty accepting limi-	2. a) describe how training will progress	2. a) by 2nd EST (6 weeks) be familiar with both objective and subjective	
	tations because he "never felt better"	emphasizing that per- formance is	responses to exercise training and begin to relate to responses in	
		gauged by responses, doing more	other situations, especially farm work b) by 3rd EST (12 weeks)	
		than pre- scribed is unwise	select an appropriate home exercise program and be prepared to	
		b) begin dis- cussion of home exercise	implement it	
		training program to be implemented		
		at approx. week 12, to reinforce that		
		dependent program and limitations		
		are only temporary		

(Patient ID Stamp) C. P.			CARDIAC REHAB CARE PLAN	
Date Identified	**Need/Problem**	**Approach**	**Behavioral Objectives**	**Date Achieved Changed**
			The patient will be able to	
	3. needs planned	3. discuss that	3. express a plan for personal	
	relaxation program	proper relaxation is as important to good health as	relaxation and describe the method chosen by 3rd EST	
		proper exercise, relaxation should also be planned		
	Educational			
	4. needs awareness of exercise principles,	4. present explanations as relevant to training	4. by the time of 3rd EST a) know his THR and accurately count his HR	
	methods, and guidelines for safe and effec-	events, conversation among patients, and	response to any exercise b) describe the frequency and duration of exercise	
	tive home training program	questions by patient	necessary to maintain fitness. c) explain how he intends	
			to perform his selected home exercise. d) state precautions	
			appropriate to his selection. e) express a commitment	
			to continuing exercise as a life-style.	

(Patient ID Stamp)

C. P.	**PHYSICIANS' ORDER SHEET**

Date/Time	ORDERS
7/11/XX 8:30 a.m.	Exercise Prescription #1
	Intensity: work to achieve progressive THR's based on 1st test MHR of 160 as follows:
	week 1-2 @ 70% = 112
	week 3-4 @ 75% = 120
	week 4-5 @ 80% = 128
	week 5-6 @ 85% = 136
	Duration: begin training time @ 20 min., progress to 30 min. by week 6, begin with short intervals of 2-3 min. each and gradually extend.
	Frequency: monitored training sessions 3X/wk.
	Type: isotonic activities, devices as available.
	Retest in 6 weeks.
	J. D., M.D.
8/25/XX (week 6)	Exercise Prescription #2
	Intensity: based on 2nd test MHR of 174 increase THR to 148 (85%)
	Increase duration to 40-45 min.
	Retest in 6 weeks.
	J. D., M. D.

(Patient ID Stamp)

C. P.

| | PHYSICIANS' ORDER SHEET |

Date/Time	ORDERS
10/8/XX (week 12)	Exercise Prescription #3
	Intensity: based on 3rd test MHR of 170 maintain THR @ 148.
	Duration may be increased to 60 min. if desired.
	Begin weaning from monitored to home program.
	Retest in 6 weeks.
	J. D., M.D.
10/20/XX (week 18)	Exercise Prescription #4
	Continue as prescription #3
	Complete transfer to independent exercise.
	Retest in 6 weeks.
	J. D., M.D.
1/5/XX (week 24)	Exercise Prescription #5
	Discharge from monitored program.
	Continue home exercise 3X/wk.
	Schedule every 3 months monitored exercise sessions
	Schedule retest in 6 months.
	J. D., m. D.

References

1. COMMITTEE on EXERCISE, *Exercise Testing and Training of Individuals with Heart Disease or at High Risk for Its Development: A Handbook for Physicians* (New York: The American Heart Association, 1975), p. 35.

2. BRUCE, R. A. and LERMAN, J., "Exercise Testing and Training in Relation to Myocardial Infarction," *Postgraduate Medicine,* April 1975, p. 64.

3. HELLERSTEIN, H. K., et al., "Principles of Exercise Prescription," *Exercise Testing and Exercise Training in Coronary Heart Disease* (New York: Academic Press, 1973), p. 139.

4. AMERICAN COLLEGE of SPORTS MEDICINE, *Guidelines for Graded Exercise Testing and Exercise Prescriptions* (Philadelphia: Lea & Febiger,, 1975), p. 41.

5. COMMITTEE on EXERCISE, *Exercise Testing and Training of Apparently Healthy Individuals: A Handbook for Physicians* (New York: The American Heart Association, 1972), p. 13.

6. ROSKAMM, H., "Optimum Patterns of Exercise for Healthy Adults," *Physical Activity and Cardiovascular Health,* March 1967, pp. 895-899.

7. MATHEWS, D. and FOX, E., *The Physiological Basis of Physical Education & Athletics* (Philadelphia: W. B. Saunders Company, 1976), pp. 245-246.

8. *Ibid.,* p. 247.

9. ASTRAND, P. O. and RODAHL, K. *Textbook of Work Physiology,* 2nd ed. (New York: McGraw-Hill Book Co., 1977), p. 295.

10. MATHEWS and FOX, *op. cit., p. 24.*

11. AMERICAN COLLEGE of SPORTS MEDICINE, *op. cit.,* p. 44.

12. COMMITTEE on EXERCISE, *Exercise Testing and Training of Individuals With Heart Disease or at High Risk for Its Development* (New York: American Heart Association, 1972), p. 25.

13. MANN, G., et al., "The Amount of Exercise Necessary to Achieve & Maintain Fitness in Adult Persons," *Southern Medical Journal,* May 1971, p. 553.

14. SIEGEL, W., BLOMQUIST, G., and MITCHELL, W. H., "Effects of a Quantitated Physical Training Program on Middle-Aged Sedentary Males," *Circulation,* Vol. 41, 1970, pp. 19-29.

15. HELLERSTEIN, *op. cot.,* p. 158.

16. COMMITTEE on EXERCISE, *op. cit.,* p. 28.

17. MANN, *op. cit.,* p. 551.

18. STOEDEFALKE, K., "Physical Fitness Programs for Adults," *The American Journal of Cardiology,* May 1974, p. 789.

19. SELYE, H., *The Stress of Life* (New York: McGraw-Hill Book Company, 1956), p. 3 and p. 47.

20. BENSON, H. *The Relaxation Response* (New York: Avon Publishers, 1975), pp. 141-149.

19

implementation of phase IV cardiac rehabilitation

Behavioral Objectives

After completion of this chapter, the reader should be able to:

■ identify the major components of a formal outpatient **cardiac rehabilitation program**.

■ list at least six program policies that can significantly **affect nursing** functions.

■ explain three common reasons for nonadherence to an **ongoing** rehab program.

■ discuss the application of Maslow's theory of behavior to motivating long-term program participation.

■ name two common side effects of exercise training **and give** possible underlying causes.

■ state potential complications due to exercise interaction **with at** least six common cardiac drugs.

■ describe a useful method for assessing chest pain as an acute change in a rehab patient's condition.

Introduction

Implementation is a dynamic part of the Phase IV nursing process. It requires awareness of the formal program structure in which the cardiac rehab nurse must function. Components of that structure help shape each patient's rehab plan and directly influence its implementation.

Implementation requires utilization of the other three elements of the nursing process—assessment, planning, and evaluation. While carrying out each patient's rehab plan, the nurse must be able to adapt her functions and coordinate the services of other team members to meet changing patient needs.

Program Formality

Ideally, the cardiac rehab nurse specialist is involved with the Phase IV outpatient program from its conception. Nursing input during research, development, organization, and installation stages of a formal outpatient program is vital to successful function.

Whether involved from the start or joining a long-standing program, the nurse needs to be familiar with program formalities. The following questions can be used as a checklist for reviewing program structure.

Philosophy and Purpose

What is the official statement? Has it been endorsed by representatives of each profession to be involved with the rehab program? Has it been discussed with staff members? Does it state the importance of nursing involvement?

The most simple, and perhaps most functional, philosophy is a statement of belief in the need for a comprehensive service that fulfills the cardiac rehabilitation definition.

Organizational Structure

What is the flow of authority governing the program? To what department or service is the program assigned? Who is responsible for the general program? For specific functions? What professional functions are inherent in the program structure? What ancillary support functions are available?

Definition of the following roles and relationships are most significant: **Medical Involvement.** Responsibility for medical supervision and general program guidance may be assigned to one physician, a rotating series of physicians, or a medical advisory committee. Administrative and advisory tasks accompanying this position directly affect the quality and success of the program. Specific responsibilities should be defined from the outset. Generally, the medical director(s) is not responsible for direct patient care.

Patients are referred to the program by their personal physicians who retain medical responsibility. Orders for program-related diagnostic studies and therapeutic interventions (such as exercise testing and training) must come from the attending physician. Frequent communication between rehab nurse and attending physician is essential to effective Phase IV care.

Other Health Professionals. The availability of other members of the health care team is essential to program effectiveness. In some cases, team members may be available on-site to provide direct patient care. In others, they may be distant resources to be consulted by the nurse when specific problems arise.

Administrative Relationships. Regardless of the type of institution in which the program functions, a manager of some type is assigned to help maintain order and flow. Selected management responsibilities may be delegated to the nurse; however, these should be defined in advance and not allowed to interfere with the nurse's primary concern—the patient. Assigning a secretary/clerk to the program to handle daily administrative tasks should be considered.

Nursing Functions. Nursing functions in the Phase IV outpatient rehab setting are described throughout Unit IV of this text. Like the roles of other professionals, a description of nursing responsibilities must be included when the program is organized (see Chapter 1 for a job description outline; see Chapter 16 for Phase IV nursing requisites).

Program Policies

What policies have been developed to guide program functions? Is there nursing representation on the policy committee? Every outpatient cardiac rehab program should have a predetermined policy on each of the following program functions.

1. Patient Referral. How will program candidates be obtained? Physician referral only? Can any physician refer?
2. Candidate Admission. What pre-admission data are required for review (history, physical exam, lab tests, and so on)? What are the criteria for exclusion? Is admission "all or none" program participation or is modified participation possible (e. g., only educational program)? Who is responsible for making the admission decision?
3. Exercise Stress Test. What pretest preparation is required for every test? What test procedures are acceptable? Who is responsible for conducting the exercise stress test? What informed consent format is to be utilized? What data collection is required routinely?
4. Exercise Prescription. Who is responsible for prescribing individual training specifications? How often is prescription update or recertification required?
5. Exercise-Training Program. What are staffing requirements for the exercise facility? Who is responsible for supervising the training program? How much flexibility is the exercise supervisor allowed in carrying out prescriptions? What informed consent format is to be utilized? Is every patient to be monitored continuously? What are specific requirements for intermittent monitoring and specific criteria for selective monitoring? What other performance checks are required? How long is the formal exercise-training program. Who is responsible for prescribing home exercise specifications?
6. Progress Review. Who is responsible for reviewing patients' progress? How often? What findings mandate more thorough evaluation? What

are criteria for discontinuing training? How often are status reports generated to the attending physician? By whom? How often will progress be evaluated by repeat exercise testing?

7. Interdisciplinary Referrals. What referrals require the attending physician's order? What interdisciplinary involvement is considered routine?

8. Patient and Family Education. How much flexibility is the nurse educator allowed? What resources and budget are available for educational purposes?

9. Complications and Side Effects. How should unusual responses be handled? Who is responsible for on-site evaluation of exercise complications? What are routine methods for treating common side effects?

10. Emergencies. What emergency equipment is required in every exercise-testing and training area? Who is responsible for assuring operational readiness? Is an emergency communication system available? What emergency training is required for staff? How often? What emergency procedures are approved for nursing staff?

11. Discharge. Who is responsible for discharging patients? What are discharge criteria? What predischarge data are required? Is there to be any postdischarge follow-up?

Operational Considerations

What routine functions are required in conjunction with program operations? Who is responsible?

Predetermination of functions in the following areas contributes to smooth operation:

1. Personnel. Is there a specific job description for each staff member? Is there a department organizational chart illustrating staff relationships? Have staffing patterns been arranged to allow optimal availability of program services?

2. Administrative. Has a fee schedule been established for program services? Have accounting, billing, and insurance services been assigned? Has clerical assistance been provided?

3. Equipment and Supplies. Who is responsible for equipment safety and function? Is a preventive maintenance program in effect? Have repair services been arranged? Who is responsible for supply inventory? Is adequate space available?

4. Forms and Records. Have appropriate flow sheets and report forms been developed for program use? Have they been reviewed and approved by the medical record committee?

Have inhouse brochures and/or instruction sheets been developed to supplement patient education? Have they been reviewed and approved by the medical education committee?

What statistics, reports, and so on are required for program analysis?

Program Procedures

What techniques have been predetermined for routine program use? Who is responsible for carrying out each procedure? Are specific instructions available?

The technical aspects of the following program functions are usually defined in procedural form (it is understood that the techniques may be interposed with professional functions):

1. Preparation of the patient preceding exercise stress testing
2. Equipment operation and data collection during an exercise test.
3. Posttest data computation and report completion.
4. Specification of exercise-training procedures is relative to the type of program, equipment available, and so on and may include description of equipment use, description of monitoring techniques, description of exercise performance sequence, and data collection and recording.

Selected professional nursing functions as discussed throughout this unit may also be outlined in procedural form.

Plan Adaptability

Implementation of a Phase IV rehab plan is not a one-time nursing function, but rather is an ongoing complex event. Implementation should be viewed as a series of adaptations to the original rehab care plan. Since outpatient rehab is a dynamic process, change is an everyday expectation. Sensitivity and flexibility are essential nursing skills for effective implementation. The nurse must identify change, sometimes subtle, sometimes dramatic, in every patient, and she must be prepared to alter her plan of care according to the change assessed.

Change is progress. And progress can be either positive or negative. The nurse must anticipate either and be prepared for both. The patient's health care progresses with changes in his health status. Some changes can be anticipated for most patients; others occur only on rare occasions.

Positive Change

Physiological improvement is a major nursing goal of Phase IV cardiac rehabilitation. As the patient progresses through his rehab plan, the nurse should be constantly looking for evidence that the desired training effects (see Chapter 16) are occurring. For example, a gradual decrease in heart rate responses to the same measured workload, or a change in attitude from depression to optimism is a sign of progress—positive change! Such observations should be documented and the patient advised of progress made. As discussed in the preceding chapter, the rate at which improvement occurs varies from patient to patient. Remember that rehabilitation is not only the achievement of selected goals, but, perhaps more important, also the maintenance of the improved health state. The maintenance of positive change would seem to be proportional to continued participation. It has been shown that patients who drop out of a rehab program experience major cardiovascular events in a significantly shorter period of time than those who remain active.[1]

Maintaining Impetus. To accomplish the physiological goals for which the Phase IV plan was designed, the patient must adhere to the exercise-training schedule. Maintaining positive direction is a continual nursing challenge throughout implementation. Common problems leading to patient attrition can frequently be anticipated by the nurse and appropriate adjustments incorporated into the rehab plan to prevent discontinuation.

Perceived "Cure." Ironically, some patients who exhibit early or dramatic improvement interpret their good fortune as total rehabilitation, closely akin to cure. This false security may lead them to the unfortunate decision that they no longer need the program. Close communication with these "super" responders may provide the nurse with clues that such a thought process is taking place. Educating the patient as to the limited value of his responses to date and re-educating him about the nature of his disease should dissuade him from believing himself to be a miracle case.

Realistic Conflicts. Long-term program compliance is frequently interrupted by the very real everyday concerns for time and money. Ideally, most Phase IV patients have returned to work or are about to. Programs that operate on a 9 A.M. to 5 P.M. daily schedule (or that meet on a 5 to 6 P.M. three-times-a-week schedule) may exclude the business commuter. If time conflicts are anticipated among the patient population, the nurse should consider suggesting to the patients involved that they discuss with their employer the possibility of having sick time off for three hours a week to keep their program appointments. Generally, this is most conveniently arranged by scheduling the patient's exercise appointment so that he arrives at work one hour late or leaves one hour early three days a week. The patient may request that the nurse intercede in discussing this possibility with his employer.

Since not all jobs are conducive to such time changes, the other consideration is to adjust program hours to accommodate availability of the majority of patients. If most patients work 8 A.M. to 4 P.M. or 9 A.M. to 5 P.M. but would be able to participate either before or after work, thought should be given to reserving early morning hours such as 6 to 10 A.M. or evening hours such as 4 to 8 P.M. for those back in the work force.

Although program scheduling is generally a matter of policy, not solely a nursing decision, the nurse is in the position to survey the time problems of her program patients, present them to the appropriate authority, and recommend remedial alternatives.

As discussed in Unit III, financial problems are not uncommon with cardiac patients. It is the nurse's responsibility to know what long-term program participation will cost a patient and what financial alternatives are available. Should an unanticipated financial problem arise at any point during program participation, such as the patient's spouse is unexpectedly laid off before the patient is able to return to work, the nurse should immediately arrange referral to the appropriate counselor or agency so that if assistance is available, it can be provided without interrupting the training program.

Enhancing Motivation. Providing exercise variety and adapting performance routines to individual interests (as discussed in the preceding chapter) will help prevent boredom. But long-term participation is largely the result of meaningful motivation. Using her knowledge of human behavior, the nurse needs to examine what stimulates each patient to participate. It should be recognized that factors affecting a patient's initial program commitment are not necessarily the same factors that will encourage him to continue over a long period of time.[2] Although many theories of human behavior could be applied to motivate the long-term cardiac rehab patient, the one that is probably most useful is Maslow's need hierarchy (see Chapter 2).[3]

Periodic identification of each patient's position relative to this hierarchy will help the nurse determine which stimulus is needed to enhance motivation. For example, initial program involvement may result from lower-level needs, such as physiological or safety concerns. Memory of the acute experience and the fear of death that accompanied it is still vivid. Return to work and the security of a weekly salary may not yet have been realized. Therefore, the patient is strongly motivated to get involved in a program that he perceives will fulfill these basic needs.

As time passes, the acute memory fades and social norms are regained. The patient will not be motivated to continue in the training program unless an attempt is made to help the patient achieve higher-level needs. Specifically, patients who are doing well and exhibiting positive change will no longer be motivated by fear or insecurity. Implementation must now focus on having the program provide social fulfillment and ego satisfaction.

While planning to meet psychosocial goals (Chapter 18), general methods for meeting higher-level needs were considered and incorporated into the rehab plan. Emphasizing the right stimulus to provide the right motivation at the right time is an implementation skill (see Table 19-1).

Table 19-1
Aids to Program Adherence

Social Motivators	Ego Motivators
Acceptance by professionals	Positive feedback by program professionals
Involvement of significant others	Verbal praise Visible reward gimmicks for successful achievements
Peer involvement	
Exercise groups Education groups Support groups	Report cards Gold stars Blue ribbons, and so on
Special events	Professionals asking for program advice, assistance or ideas
Holiday decorations and/or favors Program "graduation"	Patient-to-patient teaching Organizing group meetings or special events
"Graduate cardiac club"	

A patient's need progression does not run one way and is not stagnant. As the patient's condition and circumstances change, so too does his position in Maslow's framework. A patient who has been in the program for several weeks and has been motivated by the social contacts it provides may experience chest pain for the first time since his myocardial infarction. Interpreting the new occurrence as a survival threat, the patient out of physiological need will be motivated to adhere to any regimen directed by a health professional that has life-saving implications.

Although recognizing behavior levels and providing appropriate stimuli do not guarantee adherence, such nursing action is certainly a valuable step toward long-term compliance. Individualized motivation is a significant component of implementation.

Negative Change

Change is not limited to good news. Realizing that things can go wrong even with the best planning, the nurse must be constantly on the lookout for evidence of lack of improvement or even of decline.

Side Effects. In preceding rehab phases, the patient was taught not only the "right" things about exercise, but also the "wrong" things—the things that should be avoided and the precautions that should be taken. In helping the patient prepare for his home exercise program, precautions should be re-emphasized.

Whether in the dependent program or at home, most side effects can be minimized by adhering to basic exercise principles. Most important, insist on adequate warm-up and gradual progression. Be sure that equipment and environment are acceptable and that performance is correct.

Even when all precautions are taken, occasional side effects can occur. Early recognition and intervention are essential not only in concern for the problem at hand, but also to reduce the discouragement and frustration that accompany negative exercise experiences.

Muscular Soreness. Newcomers to exercise usually expect some degree of muscle soreness and tend to be more surprised when it doesn't happen than when it does. Patients should be routinely questioned concerning exercise tolerance. Complaints of aches and pains should not be taken lightly.

Just as exercise training is specific to the muscle groups performing the work, the type of discomfort will be specific to the type of work being performed. That is, joggers are prone to shin splints, rope jumpers to calf muscle strain, and so on.

Simple muscular soreness is a delayed reaction usually experienced several hours to a day after the activity. When it occurs, the treatment of choice is rest of the aching part. As soreness resolves, exercise may be resumed, but performance adjustment such as decreased intensity or duration, will probably be needed to avoid recurrence.

Acute Musculoskeletal Discomfort. If an exerciser presents with sudden, severe, or persistent pain in a muscle or joint, strain, sprain, or stress fracture should be suspected. The patient should be referred for medical evaluation and treatment.

Fatigue. General fatigue is a nebulous complaint difficult to assess. Many variables can contribute to a state of tiredness. In some situations, fatigue may be an expected transitory response. In others, fatigue may herald a major health concern.

When a cardiac patient complains of undue or prolonged fatigue, thorough nursing investigation is in order. Analyzing fatigue goes beyond determining the obvious sleep-wake relationship. The patient, in fact, may be tired from either too little or too much sleep. But such extremes in sleep patterns are in themselves symptoms of a greater problem, not the cause of wakeful fatigue.

The patient should be specifically questioned about recent events that may have influenced the apparent alteration in his energy state. He should also be examined for signs of change in his physiological status. Table 19-2 lists common physical and psychological factors contributing to fatigue states commonly seen in Phase IV.

Table 19-2
Common Fatigue Factors

Psychological	Physical
Emotional state	Exercise extremes
Fear	Noncompliance with prescribed regimen
Anxiety	Overexertion
Depression	
Boredom	
Work status	Work status
Awaiting return decision	Recently returned or resumed
Unable to return	full time
Tense working conditions	
Change from previous position	
Sexual activity	Sexual activity
Fear to resume	Recently resumed
Impotence	
Spouse reluctance	
	Dietary changes
	Noncompliance with prescribed regimen, for example, not restricting salt, not supplementing potassium
	Self-imposed diets
	Medications
	Noncompliance with prescribed medicine
	New medicine added recently
	Dosage of medicine changed recently
	Addition of self-prescribed medicine

Table 19-3

Potential Exercise/Drug Complications

Drug	Pharmacological Action	Exercise Physiological Action	Potential Complications
Antidysrhythmics	Suppress ectopic activity through prolongation of the refractory period; prolong QRS and QT intervals in proportion to their concentration	Exercise demands may increase irritability above drug control levels.	Dysrhythmias; masking of ischemic ECG indications
Antihypertensives	Act at various neural sites to reduce arteriolar resistance and promote vasodilatation; therefore, diastolic B/P lowers, and in turn systolic B/P lowers	Redistribution of circulation during exercise provides needed oxygen to exercising muscles through vasodilatation.	Hypotensive crisis, especially in immediate postexercise state after high-level exercise
Digitalis	Positive inotropic, increases force of contraction; decreases intracellular potassium; depresses ST segment on ECG.	Increase in stroke volume (due to increased force of contraction) is needed to increase oxygen transport.	"Digitalis effect," ST segment depression on ECG, mimics ischemic response
Diuretics	Promote loss of salt and water in fluid retaining states; frequently deplete potassium	Increased muscular action of exercise (both cardiac and skeletal) requires stable fluid and electrolyte state.	Hypokalemic dysrhythmia, muscular weakness and poor performance
Propranolol (Inderal)	A beta-adrenergic blocker—negative chronotropic (decreases heart rate) and negative inotropic (decreases force of contraction) effects reduce myocardial oxygen need.	Exercise requires increase in both heart rate and force of contraction as essential to oxygen transport.	Inadequate HR and B/P response to exercise; left ventricular failure
Long-acting nitrates	Increase venous storage capacity and, thereby, reduce work of the left ventricle with decreased myocardial oxygen demand and less chest pain	Redistribution of circulation during exercise, provides needed oxygen to exercising muscles through vasodilatation.	Hypotension (generally not as sudden or severe as may occur with antihypertensives)

If assessment of the fatigue symptom reveals a psychological problem, the rehab plan will need adjusting to provide the greater support and education indicated. If a pathological condition is suspected, the patient's physician should be contacted and appropriate medical and nursing intervention planned.

Fainting. The importance of adequate cool-down following exercise was mentioned in the preceding chapter. Extensive vasodilatation occurs during exercise to deliver needed oxygen to exercising muscles. If exercise is stopped abruptly, the muscle pump action responsible for returning venous flow ceases and venous pooling occurs. Dizziness, fainting, and a drop in blood pressure frequently accompany this alteration in circulation.

Treatment of choice is prevention. Each patient should know the importance of gradual exercise cessation to permit gradual compensatory vasocontriction. Patients should also be taught to avoid hot showers immediately after exercise since surface heat would aggravate peripheral vasodilatation and would be likely to precipitate fainting.

Should a patient faint or show other signs of venous pooling, laying him flat and elevating his legs to promote venous return is the usual remedial action. A simple venous pooling event is self-limited. No additional treatment is usually required. However, the event should be explained to the patient who may have interpreted this sudden occurrence as something more serious, such as a heart attack.

Complications. In any assembly of cardiac patients, including an outpatient cardiac rehab program, there is potential for a major health crisis to occur. Fortunately, the most serious cardiac complications, cardiac arrest and acute myocardial infarction, occur only rarely in outpatient exercise programs. In 1978, William Haskell surveyed 30 cardiac rehab programs and found 61 major cardiovascular complications in over one-and-one-half million hours of exercise participation. Fourteen events were fatal.[4]

Prevention of complications is an inherent goal of every cardiac rehab program. Frequently, signs and/or symptoms of impending problems can be identified early enough so that appropriate intervention can be undertaken and catastrophe averted. Throughout implementation, the following areas of nursing assessment and intervention are of particular concern:

Medication: Exercise Incompatibility Most nurses are aware that certain drugs used in combination with certain other drugs form an admixture and produce unexpected and sometimes disastrous results for the patient. A general analogy can be drawn between the drug-to-drug admixture and the incompatibility that occurs when certain drugs are used in combination with exercise. Drugs may inhibit or accentuate expected exercise responses. Knowing exactly what medication the patient is taking, how much, and how often is essential to assessing responses and preventing problems. A list of potential complications due to exercist-drug interaction is presented in Table 19-3.

Prescription medicines are not the only culprits to cause unusual responses or precipitate complications. Self-prescribed, over-the-counter drugs can be more troublesome than physician-prescribed properly used medicines. The possible adverse effects of something from the drugstore shelf used without awareness of exercise influence are too numerous to tabulate. Consider the possibilities with these well-known remedies: cold-allergy capsules frequently contain atropine or scopolamine; nasal decongestant sprays may contain Neo-Synephrine; "extra strength pain relievers" may contain more caffeine than several cups of coffee. When there is any suspicion about drug effects, a specific point should be made to ask the patient what drugs in addition to those prescribed by his physician he may be taking. Many patients underrate the impact of nonprescriptive drugs.

ECG Changes. Programs using continuous monitoring with exercise provide the nurse with an avenue of performance comparison and assessment—the exercise rhythm strip. It is likely that in some cases, ECG changes would be the first sign of trouble. Identification of such change and prompt follow-up has often prevented more serious complications from developing. A study by Jackson of close to 2,000 patients in a telemetry-monitored exercise-training program demonstrated that 34 percent of Phase IV rehab patients developed significant dysrhythmias at some time during exercise performance. The majority of these dysrhythmias were recorded as ventricular ectopics.[5] Chapter 20 discusses exercise ECG abnormalities.

Chest Pain. The occurrence of chest pain as a new symptom is, at least, a frightening experience for the Phase IV patient. As a progressive symptom in a previously stable angina patient, it may be referred to as pre-infarction pain. It may occur before, during, or after exercise. Once this negative change is identified, complete nursing assessment becomes the priority.

The most practical approach to assessing the chest pain problem is to follow the problem oriented outline described in Chapter 4. The use of SOAP provides a logical guide for acute symptom investigation and documentation.

To obtain subjective information, S of SOAP, a concise, specific nursing history should be taken. The following information should be solicited:

1. Location and radiation of pain. Where is the pain? Ask the patient to point to or outline the affected area.
2. Onset and precipitating factors. Does it occur suddenly or gradually? Do certain activities provoke it?
3. Duration. How long does it last?
4. Character. What does the pain feel like? Stabbing, sharp, dull, and so on?
5. Associated or accompanying symptoms. Do you experience shortness of breath, palpitations, and so on?
6. Alleviating or aggravating factors. Did drugs and/or rest relieve the pain? Does coughing, specific movements, and so on aggravate the pain?

Objective information obtained by the nurse, "O" of SOAP usually includes:

1. An abbreviated cardiovascular examination: Inspection for color, appearance, respiratory rate, and so on; auscultation for heart sounds and apical rate, lung sounds, blood pressure (both arms).
2. A 12 lead ECG.

"A" of SOAP for assessment or determination of the cause of the problem is the nursing conclusion that results from the preceding investigation. A summary outline of the more serious complications that may present with chest pain can be found in Table 19-4.

Chest pain can also be indicative of noncardiac problems, and these possibilities should not be overlooked. Gastrointestinal diseases may cause chest pain of the same type as angina pectoris. Among gastrointestinal problems encountered are esophagitis, esophageal spasm, cholecystitis, gastric ulcer, and hiatal hernia. To further confuse the pain evaluation, ECG changes can occur with some of these problems.

Musculoskeletal problems of the torso can mimic cardiac pain, but may be intensified by pressing on the affected area. This, of course, does not occur with cardiac problems.

Some patients present with typical angina pectoris, but all cardiac studies are negative. When no physical problem can be uncovered, an emotional cause should be sought. The patient's past and current mental health history is important in assessing psychological causes of pain.

Deciding appropriate nursing intervention is the immediate planning, "P" of SOAP that takes place. Should the staff cardiologist be summoned to provide acute medical care? Should the patient's physician be contacted to order further diagnostic studies for differential diagnosis? Or is a simple lesson in the proper use of nitroglycerin in order?

Full documentation of the crises just assessed and handled is a nursing responsibility. The chest pain assessment guide using the SOAP format may be a helpful recording tool as shown in Table 19-5.

Once the immediate problem is dealt with and documented, further adjustments in the total rehab plan will need to be considered. Depending upon the incident, some plan revisions may require full input of the rehab team, while others may be simple nursing adjustments. For example, will the patient's participation in the exercise program be temporarily postponed until his acute gastrointestinal problem is controlled? Is this patient a poor candidate for further exercise training, and should that portion of his rehab problem be discontinued? Should an order for pre-exercise nitroglycerin prophylaxsis be obtained?

Summary

Change in the patient means change in the nursing plan. Such change is a function of implementation.

Progress Reports

Charting progress is an outpatient cardiac rehab program, whether positive or negative, is a major implementation component. Both the chronology and the characteristics of each patient's progress are of interest.

Table 19-4

Characteristics of Cardiac-Related Complications
Commonly Presenting as Chest Pain

	Onset	Precipitating Factors	Duration	Character
Angina pectoris	Sudden or slow gradual build up	Activity, walking in cold weather, emotional upset	Less than 10 minutes	Tightness, pressure, squeezing
Prinzmetal angina	Sudden	*Not* usually associated with exercise	Usually longer than angina pectoris	Same as angina pectoris, but more intense
Pre-infarction angina (coronary insufficiency)	Sudden	May occur with little or no effort	Usually longer than angina pectoris	Same as angina but with steady increase in frequency of attacks
Myocardial infarction	Sudden	May occur at rest or with exercise	At least 30 minutes, usually one to two hours	Severe crushing, squeezing stabbing pain
Acute pericarditis	Sudden	*Not* associated with effort	Continuous, hours to days	Sharp, stabbing, or only an ache
Pulmonary embolus	Sudden	History of phlebitis	Lasts hours	Sharp stabbing pleuritic pain
Dissecting aortic aneurysm	Sudden	None	May be hours depending on how fast dissection progresses	Excrutiating chest pain, knifelike

Associated Signs and Symptoms	Relieved by	Associated ECG changes	Location	Radiation
prehension, pnea, diaphoresis al gallop (S₄)	Rest and/or nitroglycerin or similar vasodilator	May have ST depression especially with an exercise stress test, inverted T waves	Midsternal	To jaws, shoulder, arms, fingers
prehension, pnea, diaphoresis	Sometimes by NTG, but *not* by rest	Chief identifying mark of Prinzmetal is ST elevation with pain which returns to baseline when pain subsides; may have ventricular dysrhythmia with acute episode	Midsternal	May radiate to arms, shoulder, etc.
ne as angina pectoris	Increased NTG ingestion associated with attacks	Intermittent ST depression; T wave abnormalities	Midsternal	Same as angina pectoris
anosis, diaphoresis, pnea, palpitations, prehension, tricular gallop (S₃)	Narcotic analgesic	ST elevation and eventual formation of Q waves	Anterior midsternal	To jaws, shoulder, arms, back
icardial friction rub, er, pain when turn-; palpitations	ASA, Tylenol, leaning forward, sitting	Concave curvature of ST elevation lasts up to two weeks; T wave inversion lasts up to two weeks; no Q waves	Midsternal or precordial	Radiates to back; rarely to arms
anosis, dyspnea, noptysis, loud P₂, ural friction rub	Narcotic analgesic	May have Q waves; if massive PE, may have acute cor pulmonale, these changes may occur and disappear rapidly	Midsternal or lateral chest	To shoulder and neck
creased B/P in one n; aortic insufficient rmur, pulsus para-xus, cyanosis, dia-oresis pallor	Narcotic; surgery is needed	No characteristic ECG changes	Anterior midchest; pain shifts as dissection progresses	To lower back

Table 19-5
Nursing Assessment Guide for Acute Chest Pain

Subjective Information

Specific pain history
  Location and radiation
  Onset
  Duration
  Character

Precipatating factors
Associated symptoms
Alleviating factors
Aggravating factors

Objective Information

Cardiovascular exam

Inspection

  Color and appearance
  Breathing

Auscultation

  Heart sounds and apical rate
  Lung sounds
  B/P both arms

12 lead ECG

  Rate
  Rhythm
  Axis
  P waves
  QRS complex
  ST segments
  T waves

Assessment Conclusion

Compare findings to the
following possibilities

Angina pectoris
Prinzmetal angina
Pre-infarction angina
Myocardial infarction

Pericarditis
Pulmonary embolus
Aortic aneurysm
GI pathology
Musculoskeletal problem
Psychological problem

Plan

Immediate nursing intervention

  Patient care as necessary
  STAT medical intervention or

Hospital admission
Physician orders for further
diagnostic studies, medications

Per Visit

Documentation is an intrinsic part of all nursing practice. Cardiac rehab nursing requires response entries on exercise flow sheets as well as written descriptions of nursing functions performed and patient responses assessed with each rehab visit. Self-inspection of nursing records from time-to-time is helpful in maintaining quality documentation. As a check, consider the possibility that you are invited to attend an international nursing conference in an exotic foreign country. You must leave within the hour. Could a visiting cardiac rehab nurse specialist step in and care for your patients effectively solely from the information given in your nursing records?

Periodic

As the professional in charge of the program, the nurse should assume responsibility for preparing periodic progress summations to capsulize the pages of information on each patient. Progress reports every six weeks are an information service to the patient's attending physician who usually does not have frequent access to the patient's total chart. The written summary can be added to the patient's records in the physician's office for follow-up on the patient's next office visit. Narrative format, including both subjective and objective progress information is probably most useful. Cardiac rehab nurses should also be aware that an increasing number of government agencies and private insurance companies require progress reports from nurses.

Samples of both daily and periodic progress reports are included in the case illustration at the end of this chapter.

(Patient ID Stamp)

C. P.	**CARDIAC REHAB** **PROGRESS NOTES**

Date/Time	PROGRESS NOTES
7/14/XX 9 a.m.	First exercise training session Phase IV:
	S. Patient stated he's "glad to finally be doing more work." Asking other patients about their heart attacks.
	O. HR responses on target after minor load adjustments. No ECG abnormalities. Instructed on how to operate treadmill, bicycle ergometer, arm ergometer, wall pulleys. Will review again next session.
	A. 1st exercise training session tolerated well physically and provided psychological lift.
	P. Continue training increasing performance per prescription.
	C. R., R.N.

(Patient ID Stamp)

C. P.	CARDIAC REHAB PROGRESS NOTES

Date/Time	PROGRESS NOTES
8/10/XX 9 a.m.	S. Asking about "how much better" he'll do on his 2nd EST in 2 weeks. Advised
	that training has improved his work performance over past several weeks
	and that such improvement will be reflected in test. Asked patient if he
	thought about relaxation discussion of last session—stated he thinks he can
	relax just as easily watching T.V. than some other way.
	O. Rare VPC @ rest, none with exercise. Workloads increased several times to
	maintain THR.
	A. Wife along to observe session. Seemed surprised at performance ability of
	some patients. Doing well, but still anxious to do more. Will resume teaching
	full time next month—now enjoys doing all own farm work.
	P. Ask physician to reinforce need for not "overdoing" at time of 2nd EST. *C. R., R. n.*
8/22/XX 6 a.m.	S. Patient said he'd "like to try jogging" for home exercise since he lives on a
	farm and has a lot of space good for running. Pros/cons of jogging discussed
	in detail.
	O. B/P slightly elevated today. Had to rush to get here on time due to teachers'
	meeting after school.
	A. Exercise ECG remains stable. Tolerates increased interval time well on leg
	devices.
	P. Will pursue jogging plans and discuss a bad weather alternative. *P. 9., R. n.*

Name ___C. P.___ Phase ___IV___

Date/Time		Pre-exercise			1	2
7/14/XX 8 a.m.	**HR** 74	**Rhythm** NSR	**BP** 132/84	**Device** **Load**	treadmill 3 mph 5%	wall pulleys 2 lbs. each
Program Week 1	**HR Guide** target 112		**Rx Date** 7/11/XX	**Time**	3	3
				HR peak	114	107
	HR	**Rhythm**	**BP**	**Device** **Load**	1	2
Program Week	**HR Guide**		**Rx Date**	**Time**		
				HR peak		
8/10/XX 8 a.m.	**HR** 82	**Rhythm** NSR rare VPC	**BP** 126/80	**Device** **Load**	arm ergometer 150 KPM	treadmill 3.5m 10%
Program Week 4	**HR Guide** targer 128		**Rx Date** 7/11/XX	**Time**	4½	4½
				HR peak	120	130
	HR	**Rhythm**	**BP**	**Device** **Load**	1	2
Program Week	**HR Guide**		**Rx Date**	**Time**		
				HR peak		
9/22/XX 5 p.m.	**HR** 84	**Rhythm** NSR	**BP** 140/84	**Device** **Load**	bike ergometer 600 KPM	arm ergometer 450 KPM
Program Week 9	**HR Guide** targer 148		**Rx Date** 8/25/XX	**Time**	10	5
				HR peak	150	156
	HR	**Rhythm**	**BP**	**Device** **Load**	1	2
Program Week	**HR Guide**		**Rx Date**	**Time**		
				HR peak		

Physician _____ J. D. _____

Exercise Intervals				Post-exercise		
3 bike ergometer 150 KPM	4 arm ergometer 75 KPM	5 treadmill 3mph 5%	6 wall pulleys 2 lbs. each	**HR** 85	**Rhythm** NSR	**BP** 126/80
3	3	3	3	**Total Time** 18′		**Supervised By** _C.R., R.N._
116	112	110	108			
3	4	5	6	**HR**	**Rhythm**	**BP**
				Total Time		**Supervised By**
3 wall pulleys 6 lbs. each	4 bike ergometer 450 KPM	5 arm ergometer 150 KPM	6 treadmill 3.5m 10%	**HR** 90	**Rhythm** NSR No ectopics	**BP** 130/78
4½	4½	4½	4½	**Total Time** 27′		**Supervised By** _C.R., R.N._
125	126	124	128			
3	4	5	6	**HR**	**Rhythm**	**BP**
				Total Time		**Supervised By**
3 treadmill 4mph 10%	4 wall pulleys 10 lbs. each	5 bike ergometer 600 KPM	6	**HR** 96	**Rhythm** NSR	**BP** 138/80
10	5	10		**Total Time** 40′		**Supervised By** _P.T. R.N._
145	140	142				
3	4	5	6	**HR**	**Rhythm**	**BP**
				Total Time		**Supervised By**

August 26, XXXX

Dr. D. D.
456 Center Avenue
Metropolis, U.S.

Dear Dr. D.:

Your patient, C. P., has been a participant in the Phase IV rehab program for six weeks. The following is a summation of his progress during that time:

Subjective Responses

Patient states he is able to do more with less fatigue since starting training and that he "feels better" in general. He attends training sessions faithfully and demonstrates a determined attitude to do what is in the best interest of his health.

Objective Responses

Patient has been able to progressively increase his levels of work performance. Early training effects are evidenced by decreased heart rate and blood pressure responses to his second exercise stress test performed yesterday. ECG has remained stable, with only a rare VPC.

C. P. will continue his monitored training sessions three times a week for six additional weeks per prescription of Dr. J. D. During that time, planning for the patient's home exercise training program will proceed.

A third exercise stress test is scheduled for six weeks from now to evaluate the patient's status. If responses at that time are satisfactory, the patient will begin gradual transfer to his selected home program.

I would be pleased to discuss this patient's rehabilitation program with you in detail at your convenience.

Sincerely,

C. P., R.N.
Cardiac Rehab Nurse-Specialist

References

1. BRUCE, E. H., et al., "Comparison of Active Participants and Dropouts in Cardio-pulmonary Rehabilitation Programs," *American Journal of Cardiology*, Vol. 37, January 1976, pp. 53-60.
2. HEINZELMANN, F., "Social & Psychological Factors That Influence the Effectiveness of Exercise Programs," *Exercise Testing and Exercise Training in Coronary Heart Disease* (New York: Academic Press, 1973), pp. 275-280.
3. MASLOW, A. H., *Motivation & Personality*, 2nd Ed. (New York: Harper & Row, Publishers, Inc., 1970).
4. HASKELL, W. L., "Cardiovascular Complications during Exercise Training of Cardiac Patients," *Circulation*, Vol. 57, No. 5, May 1978, pp. 920-924.
5. JACKSON, F., "The Incidence of Arrhythmia in a Cardiac Rehabilitation Exercise Program", (abstract) *American Journal of Cardiology*, January 1976, p. 144.

20

evaluation
of phase IV
cardiac
rehabilitation

Behavioral Objectives

After completion of this chapter, the reader should be able to:

- describe the expected heart rate and ECG response to exercise training.
- list at least six causes of abnormal heart rate response during training and six causes of abnormal ECG responses.
- identify ischemic ST segments on exercise rhythm strips.
- name three response comparisons to be evaluated with serial testing and give an example of training effectiveness with each.
- draft a basic plan for reviewing Phase IV program effectiveness.
- list at least six patient outcomes to be expected from an effective Phase IV program.
- explain four purposes of a discharge interview.

Introduction

To determine if assessment was accurate, planning proficient, and implementation efficient, evaluation is essential. Evaluation includes assessing current activities and looking at past events, investigating written reports, and soliciting spoken opinions, isolating individual instances and broadening the view to include the program as an entity. The nurse is responsible for evaluating the effectiveness of the health care she provides and the program in which she practices.

Evaluation of Patient Responses

Continuous Assessment

The main purpose of professional supervision of exercise training is response determination—identification of responses that occur and awareness of their significance. Seeing the patient three times a week for exercise training provides the opportunity for ongoing evaluation. Each time the patient is seen, his responses are identified, documented, and interpreted by the nurse. Response parameters generally assessed can be divided into two categories.

Subjective. How does the patient feel? How does he perceive his rehab progress and his general state of health? This information can be elicited through casual conversation rather than the monotony of a sterile "and how are you feeling today?" inquiry. Good rapport and open communication frequently produce this information spontaneously. Should the patient have a subjective complaint, thorough nursing assessment is in order and may include solicitation of specific subjective information (see Chapter 19).

Of course, subjective assessment is also concerned with what is happening in the patient's mind as well as in his body. Is he happy with his progress? Is he angry because of restrictions imposed? Is he fearful? Frustrated? The nurse may infer the presence of an emotional concern from the patient's conversation. Further dialogue might be needed to identify the exact problem.

Identifying and documenting emotional concerns as part of subjective evaluation is important in evaluating overrall health progress. Anxiety over return to work could be the cause of accelerated heart rate responses. Depression over forced retirement could be the reason for noncompliance to a medication regimen.

The frequencey of three times per week for a 12-week training program means that the nurse will become very familiar with her patients. In a sense, the nurse becomes the patient's "captive audience." The nurse cannot be expected to personally like every patient, but she is expected to give her professional best to each individual. At times, this may require conscious effort when it comes to subjective evaluation. Being able to hear what a patient is telling you, even when you think you've heard it ten times before, can be the biggest communication challenge of cardiac rehab.

Objective. Selected physical parameters, representative of the general health state of the patient, are measured with each exercise performance. The nurse supervising the exercise session is responsible not only for collecting and documenting the routine measurements, but also for recognizing the significance of the data both as a single occurrence and as a trend in the patient's health status. *Heart Rate.* As described in Chapter 18, heart rate is the major exercise guideline. In each exercise session, the exercise supervisor assists the patient to achieve his prescribed training heart rate. If interval exercise is used, the heart rate is checked during each work interval and the levels of work adjusted as necessary to maintain the desired rate for the remainder of the interval. If continuous exercise is utilized, the heart rate should be checked every two to three minutes to assure stabilization.

Assuming that no heart rate abnormality was diagnosed with the most recent exercise test, that exercise is performed correctly, and that appropriate work level adjustments are made, heart rates measured during the session should consistently be in the prescribed training range.

The occurrence of an unexpected heart rate response, either too high or too low, is considered abnormal for the session and requires that the cause be investigated. Some of the more common causes of unusual heart rate responses are presented in Table 20-1.

Table 20-1
Factors Influencing Heart Rate Response to Exercise Training

Excessive response
  Emotional states (anxiety, anger, fear)
  Low-grade fever (cold, flu, virus)
  Fatigue
  Caffeine (coffee, tea, cola)
  Nicotine
  Drugs (prescribed or over-the-counter stimulant containing compounds)
  Ischemic tachydysrhythmias
  Early pump failure
Deficient response
  Drugs propranolol (Inderal)
  Sinus node dysfunction
  Ischemic bradydysrhythmias

An important distinction needs to be made between the gradual heart rate change that is a sign of training effects and the one-time abnormal responses reviewed above. As conditioning occurs, the heart rate is expected to decrease when the *same* level of work is performed. For example, during six successive exercise sessions, a patient walks on a treadmill at 3 m.p.h./6 percent grade and demonstrates a heart rate of 150 to 156 (within the prescribed training range). During the next three sessions, he shows a heart rate decline with the same treadmill performance: session #7 HR 148, #8 HR 145, #9 HR 144. Such response indicates that the patient has become conditioned at that level of work. In order for training to progress on that piece of exercise equipment, the work level needs to be increased to bring the heart rate back into the training range.

Exercise ECG. The use of telemetry monitoring with an exercise-training program provides the nurse with two immediate evaluation advantages: continuous heart rate measurement, and constant visualization of cardiac electrical activity. The most obvious use of exercise monitoring is to allow identification of extreme rhythm changes that require emergency intervention. Fortunately, such occurrences are rare in a controlled exercise setting (see Chapter 19).

In fact, it is in identifying changes before they reach a threatening level that exercise telemetry proves its value. Heart rate can be obtained by means other then telemetry. But the fact that a heart rate is within a prescribed response range does not guarantee that the patient's ECG is normal.

The "normal" exercise ECG shows a sinus tachycardia. Normal heart rate responses during training can be as high as 160 to 170 beats per minute. A change in rhythm, conduction, or configuration of the ECG is not detectable through heart rate measurement alone. Related symptoms may be a late indicator of ECG abnormalities. Use of exercise ECG monitoring provides a means of intercepting problems.

The term "exercise ECG" as used in this discussion is synonymous with telemetry rhythm strip. Recordings pertain to single-lead tracings (as suggested in Chapter 14), and should not be confused with the modified 12 lead ECG used for exercise testing (see Chapter 17).

1. Ventricular ectopic activity. As in most cardiac settings, ventricular ectopics are the most commonly seen ECG abnormality. Nursing assessment of VPCs in the Phase IV patient is also much the same as in other cardiac settings: How frequent are the ectopics? From how many foci? What is the coupling interval?

   Should the VPCs be frequent, multifocal, have short coupling intervals, or occur in runs of three or more beats, they are a threat to the patient and immediate medical intervention should be sought.

   In an exercise setting, factors in addition to the above determinations enter into the nursing assessment of VPCs. Namely, the comparison of VPC activity at rest and with exercise. If prior to an exercise session, a patient displays occasional VPCs that are unifocal and has no other signs or symptoms of cardiac difficulty, the training program is usually conducted as planned, and the ectopic activity is carefully observed. As the heart rate increases in response to the exercise, the VPCs may completely disappear. This effect seems to be due to the change in refractory time with increased rate blocking the ectopic impulse.[1] Such VPCs are generally not worrisome because they are not usually associated with cardiac pathology.

   Conversely, should the VPCs increase in response to exercise, it is believed that underlying ischemia is usually present.[2] Progression of coronary artery disease is a possibility and, therefore, the patient should be referred to his physician for further diagnostic evaluation (see Figure 20-1).

2. Conduction defects. The occurence of widened QRS complex with exercise presents assessment challenge. With the single-lead strip generated by telemetry, it is difficult to differentiate between the

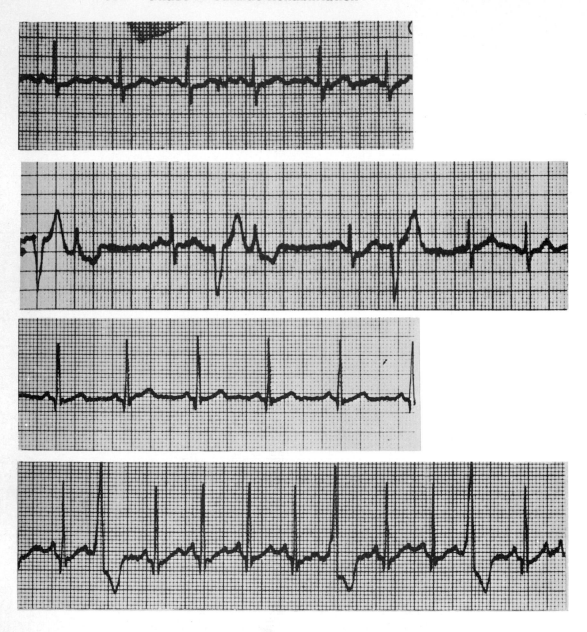

Figure 20-1. Exercise-induced ventricular ectopics. Top two strips: Pre-exercise HR 85, NSR; exercise HR 100, multiple ectopics. Bottom two strips: Pre-exercise HR 80, NSR; exercise HR 125, frequent ectopics.

widened, regular QRS of ventricular tachycardia and an alteration in intraventricular conduction producing intermittent bundle branch block. Further compounding the interpretation problem is the rapid rate resulting from exercise.

Regardless of which rhythm abnormality is suspected, a change this dramatic means that the exercise should be stopped immediately and a 12 lead ECG recorded as quickly as possible to aid diagnosis. Symptoms may or may not accompany either abnormality. The initial concern for distinction is the fact that one problem is more immediately life threatening than the other.

Intermittent bundle branch block may be rate-related with the conduction change due to arrival of the impulse while one of the bundle branches is still refractory.[3] The occurrence of a bundle branch block pattern with exercise when QRS duration was normal at rest, may or may not be pathologic.[4] However, in known cardiac patients, myocardial ischemia should be suspected as the underlying cause until medical investigation proves otherwise. As heart returns to the resting level, the block disappears (see Figure 20-2).

3. Configuration. Assessment of the ST segment is a routine part of analyzing every exercise ECG. Chapter 17 illustrated the ST assessment sequence. The nurse supervising exercise training must be aware of the implications of ST segment changes.

As with any major ECG change related to exercise, ST segment alteration raises suspicion of new or progressing cardiac pathology.

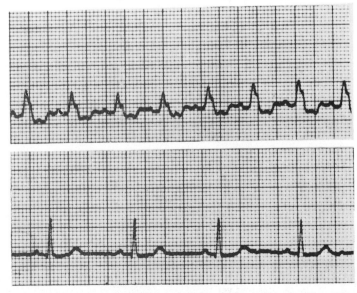

Figure 20-2. Exercised-induced conduction defect. (Top) Pre-exercise: HR 70, NSR normal conduction. (Bottom) Exercise: HR 130 (fifth interval), rate-related conduction defect.

Assuming that the telemetry frequency from which the recording is made is of diagnostic range, ST depression that is 1 mm. or greater after 80 milliseconds is representative of myocardial ischemia. But the conclusion that ST depression is ischemic should be a logical not an automatic label. There are conditions and circumstances other than coronary artery disease that can produce ST depression (see Table 20-2). Although more often encountered in the exercise-testing setting where performance and heart rates are taken to higher levels, these influences should be reviewed and discounted before an ischemic conclusion is made in evaluating ST segment depression as a new occurrence with exercise training (see Figure 20-3).

The first assumption on seeing acute ST elevation with exercise is, of course, myocardial infarction, usually corroborated by other familiar signs and symptoms. During exercise training, acute myocardial infarction is rare (see Chapter 19). The ST elevation can be a rare form of ischemic manifestation, such as with Prinzmetal's angina or may be a mirror image of a depression in an opposite lead.[5] Another underlying possibility when ST elevation occurs with exercise is the presence of ventricular aneurysm.[6]

Documentation of both subjective and objective evaluation with each rehab visit is part of the nurse's progress note (see Chapter 19). Additionally, selected exercise ECG strips are mounted as part of the exercise record.

Serial Comparison

Cardiovascular adaptation to exercise training is best evaluated by comparing the results of successive exercise tests. Improvement in systemic oxygen transport capability, as well as reduction in myocardial oxygen need, is reflected in several test parameters. Comparison of data from a recent test to data of preceding tests suggests the extent of improvement that has occurred. For such comparisons to be valid, the test must be conducted in exactly the same manner each time.

Since the degree of physiological change associated with exercise is variable, a "normal" rate or amount of improvement is not available as a standard for comparison. Adaptation is relative only to each individual. Thus, the need for frequent serial comparisons to gauge progress.

Parameters most useful for the nurse to evaluate with each cardiac rehab patient are heart rate, systolic blood pressure, and functional capacity.

Heart Rate Comparisons. In programs where serial testing is done every six weeks, most patients will show a measureable decrease in resting heart rate and submaximal work level heart rates from their pretraining test to their six-week test to their twelve-week test.

Systolic Blood Pressure Comparisons. Progressive decrease in systolic blood pressure response should also be evidenced from test to test. As training continues and the patient approaches his optimal physical state, response differences will grow less dramatic and will eventually "level-off" at an optimal level of conditioning that, impressive though it may be, requires continued training to maintain.

Table 20-2
ST Segment Mimics of Ischemia

Anemia
Carbohydrate ingestion
Cardiac abnormalities
  Left bundle branch block
  Left ventricular hypertrophy
  Pericardial disease
  Valve disease
  Wolf Parkinson-White Syndrome
Drugs
  Digitalis
  Diuretics
Hormones
Hyperventilation
Hypokalemia

An alternate method of evaluating heart rate and systolic blood pressure responses simultaneously is to compute the "double product" (see Chapter 16) and compare successive test changes. Just as each double product factor should decrease with training, the double product should be less with each additional test computation.

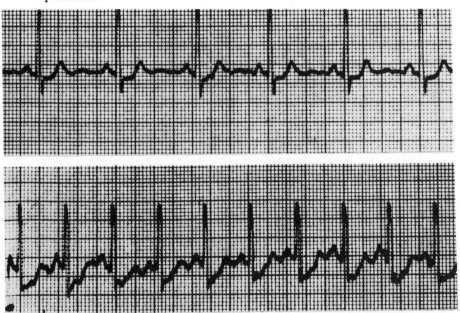

Figure 20-3. Exercise-induced ST segment depression. (Top) Pre-exercise: HR 75, NSR. (Bottom) Exercise: HR 124 (fourth interval) ST depression of 3 to 4 mm.

Functional Capacity. As the patient progresses through the training program, work tolerance improves in relation to both muscular and cardiovascular training. With each successive test, the patient should be able to perform more work. Noting the peak work performance is as important to the patient's psychosocial health progression as to the physical. If the patient is waiting to return to work, to resume softball with the neighborhood team, or to take his wife square dancing, a few levels of work can make a big difference.

In addition to indicating progress-to-date, data obtained by serial measurement are used to adjust the patient's exercise prescription after each test. For example, if the previously prescribed training heart rate was based on a peak heart rate response of 140 and the patient achieved a peak rate of 165 with the current test, the training heart rate range should be adjusted accordingly.

Rather than showing an improved performance on a second, third, or fourth test, an occasional patient will show a decline in performance capability, and/or an increase in heart rate or blood pressure response. Most often, a high degress of backsliding is the result of progressing disease. Further medical evaluation and intervention are indicated.

Program Review

Long-term care such as outpatient cardiac rehabilitation requires periodic evaluation to assure that health care provided to participants is appropriate and effective. Planned program review is an essential part of evaluation in every health care setting.

Government regulations, inspection agency guidelines, insurance company requirements, and institutional policies require that the need for continuing a long-term program be re-affirmed periodically. Frequency and type of documentation required vary. In general, serial exercise testing and nursing progress summaries every six weeks provide sufficient documentation of the extent of progress and the need for continuation of program participation to achieve objectives. Should test data and progress reports indicate that all rehab objectives have been met, discharge should be considered.

In addition to the above reviews built into the basic training plan for each patient, the quality of the program should be evaluated by the professionals involved. Formal audit procedures are utilized in most institutions and may be directly applicable to the Phase IV rehab program. Where concurrent audit procedures are not available, the nurse coordinator should initiate development of some method of program review. The following suggestions may be helpful.

The Advisory Committee of the outpatient rehab program should be asked to formulate a review policy specifying the frequency of review conferences and the professionals to be involved. A conference time and location should then be selected for convenience and consistency, for example, the first Friday of each month from 11 A.M. to noon in the exercise unit conference room.

Next, the review procedures should be defined by the appointed review committee. For instance, two categories of review might routinely be included at each conference.

Implementation Problems

The Special Event. This category would include presentation and discussion of cases in which special events such as major side effects, complications, or unusual responses have occurred. The nature of these cases probably would have required immediate nursing and/or medical intervention. Review is done here to ascertain the effectiveness of health care rendered.

The Difficult Adjustment. In this group would be presentation and discussion of cases in which implementation of the rehab plan appears ineffective. In such cases, the nurse may be unable to isolate the cause of the apparent unresponsiveness and/or may have depleted her usual exercise adjustment repertoire and may be in need of additional advice or special ideas. Professional brainstorming frequently provides the needed remedy.

Random Case Review

A number of patient charts, perhaps a predetermined percentage of the total number of program patients, are selected at random from the current files and reviewed for evidence of effective rehab care.

In a young program, the review may be a simple accounting of services performed or behaviors observed. Such gathering of information will help the review committee identify program "norms" which, as experience grows, may be refined into audit criteria. For example, of the charts reviewed, what percentage of those patients' spouses accompanied patients to the rehab unit during the first program month? If findings are consistently low, a recommendation may be that the nurse should call the spouses of new patients and extend a professional invitation for their participation in the rehab program. This observation may subsequently be assigned under a review category "involvement and support of significant others" with the criteria stating the patient's spouse should be contacted by the nurse within the first three to four weeks of the program.

Documentation

Minutes should be kept of the proceedings of the review meeting and a summary written on the chart of each patient whose case is reviewed, noting recommendations made and the disposition chosen. This disposition may be a simple suggestion that the nurse can implement or an unanticipated major decision, such as discontinuing the patient's exercise program. In either case, the patient, as an active member of the health team, is subsequently informed of the reasons for the recommended change. When major changes are involved, alternatives need to be reviewed with the patient, objectives revised, and the rehab plan changed accordingly.

Programs with access to computerized data storage and retrieval will find that the possibilities for programming checks and balances to aid auditing, counts and subcounts to profile the patient population, and plots and curves to follow program patients as a collective entity are endless.

Phase IV Termination

Discharge from an outpatient unit is the culmination of all phases of a comprehensive cardiac rehab program for it implies that the patient graduate is ready, willing, and able to take over responsibility for his cardiac health. Undoubtedly, the patient has worked hard preparing for this time. Recognition of his success by all health professionals involved will add ego strength and motivational impetus for the patient to continue his health pursuits.

Outcome Evaluation

Discharge is the collaborative decision of nurse, physician and other health professionals actively involved with the patient's rehab care. The discharge decision requires review and evaluation of the patient's behavioral accomplishments to determine to what extent Phase IV objectives have been met. Although discharge consideration generally coincides with completion of a structured exercise program, professional decision, not a calendar date, determines the actual time of discharge.

In planning Phase IV care, common nursing goals provided a generalized reference for development of individualized objectives. Common patient outcomes for Phase IV provide a related reference that can be useful for predischarge evaluation (see Table 20-3).

Table 20-3
Common Patient Outcomes for Phase IV Cardiac Rehabilitation

Physiological Outcomes

Upon discharge from the Phase IV outpatient program, the cardiac patient should be able to:

Demonstrate improved cardiovascular performance through a decrease in heart rate, systolic blood pressure, and double product when serial test results are compared.

Describe his level of physical function and explain the rationale for continuing training efforts.

Psychosocial Outcomes

Upon discharge from the Phase IV outpatient program, the cardiac patient should be able to:

Express an optimistic attitude about his health status.

Exhibit a desire to continue to pursue healthful living.

Demonstrate increasing stability in home, work, and social relationships.

Educational Outcomes

Upon discharge from the Phase IV outpatient program, the cardiac patient should be able to:

Discuss his home exercise program and describe correct application of his individualized exercise guidelines.

List his remaining risk factors and describe his plans for modification or control.

State his arrangement for professional follow-up.

The dynamic nature of cardiac rehabilitation means that a patient's objectives may be accomplished, deleted, or changed at any time during Phase IV participation. Actual rehab success is measured by the extent of achievement of Phase IV objectives. It is not expected that every patient will achieve every objective in the specified time period. Common outcomes suggest a direction of behavioral change that should occur in most patients prior to Phase IV discharge. They are a general summation of expected rehab results.

Through review of the rehab care plan, progress notes, flow sheets, test reports, and other chart information, the discharge evaluation team should be able to identify which objectives have been met and to what extent and which objectives have not been met and why. If the reviewers conclude that discharge is appropriate at this time, the recommendation is discussed with the patient and his family for final decision.

Discharge Interview

Beginning with his admission interview, the Phase IV patient has been actively involved as a member of the rehab team. Phase IV planning and implementation have revolved around discharge preparation. As part of his involvement in his own health care, the patient as a team member should also be involved in the discharge decision.

A discharge meeting should be arranged to include the patient, his significant others, and the nurse. The following items of business should be covered.

Review of Objectives. The nurse should review each objective with the patient showing objective evidence of accomplishment, such as exercise data, progress notes, and so on and requesting the patient's subjective opinion as to whether or not the extent of accomplishment met his expectations. Objectives not met should be discussed and planning for future achievement begun.

Postdischarge Health Care. The patient should be asked to describe his health care plans. Although many specifics of self-care were planned with the patient in recent weeks, feedback from the patient at this point will help the nurse identify any last minute weak spots or doubtful areas.

Arrangements for professional follow-up should be discussed at this time. Has the patient arranged an appointment with his physician, his nurse, the rehab unit, the cardiac clinic? Are other health resources needed?

Questions and Verbalization. The patient or a family member may have questions that still need to be answered or areas of concern that require clarification. They should be encouraged to ask their questions and to express their feelings about their rehab experience.

Discharge Acceptance. At the conclusion of the discharge interview, the patient should be asked if he agrees that he is ready for discharge. If he approves, a "graduation date" is chosen. If the patient feels he is not ready, his reasons are documented, new objectives are determined, and plans are made for their accomplishments.

(Patient ID Stamp)

C. P.

CARDIAC REHAB PROGRESS NOTES

Date/Time	PROGRESS NOTES
1/7/XX 1:30 p.m.	Discharge interview with patient and wife. Phase IV summary:
	Objectives accomplished as indicated on the Rehab Plan with the exception of a specific relaxation program which the patient feels he doesn't need.
	S. Both patient and wife expressed satisfaction with program results. Patient, "wouldn't have gone back to farming without knowing what I could do." Wife, program "helped relieve nervousness." Both are committed to patient continuing new healthful habits.
	O. Substantial improvement in all objective performance parameters over six month training period. Decreased HR and B/P response at rest and with submaximal work. Increase in work capacity and endurance. Exercise ECG stable throughout training.
	A. Effective rehab program meaningful to patient.
	P. Patient to continue fitness maintenance through home exercise program alternating outdoor jogging/indoor stationary bike using THR @ 150. Monitored exercise "check-up" scheduled for 3 months. Open invitation to call or visit at any time.
	C. R., R. n.

Discharge Documentation

The nurse is responsible for preparing the discharge summary following the team and patient meetings. Sufficient explanation should be provided in the written report so that it is self-contained recap of the Phase IV program. A health professional reading this one report from the patient's records should have a good overview of the health care that has transpired during the weeks of Phase IV. The format suggested in Table 20-4 provides this information in a concise, organized manner.

Table 20-4
Discharge Summary Format

I. Outcomes of Phase IV rehab care
  A. Objectives achieved
      (List objectives and abbreviate evidence of accomplishment)
  B. Objectives remaining
      (List objectives and indicate deterrants to accomplishment)
II. Summary of Phase IV
  A. Subjective progress
      (The patient's attitudes, feelings, and so on at program initiation, while in progress, and at termination)
  B. Objective progress
      (Comparison of data and measurements initially, in progress, and at termination)
  C. Nurse's summary
      (Professional opinion of program effectiveness with this patient)
  D. Patient's postdischarge health plan
      (Summarize patient's plans as discussed in the interview; include names of health professionals to be involved with future health care, send copies of this summary)

An accesory item of documentation, useful in evaluating overall program effectiveness, is the postdischarge program evaluation. A survey questionnaire could be mailed to the patient following discharge. Questionnaire structure should be such that it helps identify program strengths and weaknesses. For example, questions may be asked about educational materials utilized, exercise methods employed, attitudes of personnel, and so on. Anonymity will usually encourage more objective answers.

References

1. ELLESTAD, M. H., *Stress Testing, Principles and Practice* (Philadelphia: F. A. Davis Company, 1975) p. 148.
2. *Ibid.*, p. 150.
3. MARRIOTT, H. J. L., *Practical Electrocardiography*, 5th ed. (Baltimore, Maryland: Williams & Wilkins, 1972), p.81.
4. ELLESTAD, *op. cit.*, p. 131.
5. KALTENBACH, M., *Exercise Testing of Cardiac Patients* (Baltimore, Maryland: Williams & Wilkins, 1976), p. 82.
6. ELLESTAD, *op. cit.*, p. 120.

index

Page numbers in italics indicate figures.